D0024098

Review of Research in Nursing Education Volume VII

Kathleen R. Stevens, EdD, RN, CS
Editor

NLN Press ● New York
Pub. No. 19-6711

ISBN 0-88737-671-1

The views expressed in this publication represent the views of the authors and do not necessarily reflect the official views of the National League for Nursing.

This book was set in Garamond by Publications Development Company. The editor was Maryan Malone.

Printed in the United States of America

EDITORIAL REVIEW BOARD

iii

Cont 1/16/96

FEB 05 1996

CONTRIBUTING AUTHORS

Patricia Bailey, EdD, RN, CS
Associate Professor of Nursing
Department of Nursing
University of Scranton
Scranton, PA 18510-4595

Dona Rinaldi Carpenter, EdD, RN, CS
Associate Professor of Nursing
Department of Nursing
University of Scranton
Scranton, PA 18510

Betsy Frank, PhD, RN
Associate Professor
School of Nursing
Indiana State University
Terre Haute, IN 47809

Ruth Ann B. Fulton, DNSc, RN
Associate Professor
Nursing Program
College Misericordia
Dallas, PA 18612

Judith A. Halstead, DNS, RN
Assistant Professor of Nursing
School of Nursing
University of Southern Indiana
Evansville, IN 47712

Elizabeth Kelly, PhD, RN
Assistant Professor
College of Nursing
Texas Woman's University,
Houston Center
Houston, TX 77030

Cecile A. Lengacher, PhD, RN
Associate Professor
College of Nursing
University of South Florida
Tampa, FL 33612-4799

Marilyn H. Oermann, PhD, RN, FAAN
Associate Professor and Director of
Curriculum and Instruction
College of Nursing
Wayne State University
Detroit, MI 48202

Anne Young, EdD, RN
Associate Professor
College of Nursing
Texas Woman's University, Houston
Center
Houston, TX 77030

PREFACE

Research is fundamental to excellence in the preparation of those who would practice nursing. To this end, the National League for Nursing Council for Research in Nursing Education (CRNE) presents *Volume VII* of the *Review of Research in Nursing Education* series.

Begun in 1986, the *Review* series presents summary and analysis of educational research literature on specific topics. Through this dissemination of research, the Council wishes to influence faculty, students, and programs to strive for maximum relevance to the profession and to health care.

Volume VII presents a variety of topics. The first chapter sets the stage for continued transformation of nursing education to meet changing societal context by presenting models for nursing education. In the second chapter, this theme of changing expectations is carried through in a unique approach to analyzing research related to role theory, specifically, role stress, strain, and anxiety perceived by faculty and students. As the stage is set for education and role, the third chapter examines the significance of student faculty interactions in nursing education. The fourth chapter revisits research on the core of nursing education—teaching in the clinical setting—and provides an update on this topic. Chapter 5 is devoted to summarizing what is known about spirituality and nursing education. The last two chapters focus on the outcomes of nursing education programs. In Chapter 6, patterns of master's and doctoral program graduates generate a discussion of implications for curricula. The final chapter adds to and extends previous discussions of predictors of success on the Registered Nurse licensure examination.

The volume is a collective work of authors who sought to share their analyses with their colleagues. Their commitment to excellence is evident. It is hoped that these efforts will enhance the educational endeavors of nurse faculty and students of professional education.

Each chapter underwent careful peer review by members of the Editorial Review Board. These Board members generously shared their expertise during the review process and provided valuable guidance, for which both this editor and the authors are thankful.

The membership of the CRNE acknowledges the contribution of Dr. Florence Bourcier, RN, Associate Professor of Nursing, to the advancement of nursing education. Her untimely death is a loss to the profession.

Inquiries, letters of interest, or outlines for future chapter submissions may be directed to:

Kathleen R. Stevens, EdD, RN, CS
Editor

CONTENTS

1. **Models of Nursing Education for the Twenty-First Century**   **1**
    Elizabeth Kelly and Anne Young

2. **Role Strain, Roll Stress, and Anxiety in Nursing Faculty and Students: Theory and Research Analysis**   **40**
    Cecile A. Lengacher

3. **The Significance of Student-Faculty Interactions**   **67**
    Judith A. Halstead

4. **Research on Teaching in the Clinical Setting**   **91**
    Marilyn H. Oermann

5. **Spirituality and Nursing Education**   **127**
    Ruth Ann B. Fulton

6. **Utilization of Master's and Doctoral Program Graduates: Implications for Curricula**   **148**
    Betsy Frank

7. **Predicting Success on the Registered Nurse Licensure Examination: Past, Present, and Future**   **176**
    Dona Rinaldi Carpenter and Patricia Bailey

Chapter One

MODELS OF NURSING EDUCATION FOR THE TWENTY-FIRST CENTURY

Elizabeth Kelly, PhD, RN
Anne Young, EdD, RN

Professional nursing practice is changing at an unprecedented rate. Health care reform is shifting the focus of practice from institution to community, from acute care to prevention (Oermann, 1994). Expanding technologies have caused the lifespan to increase, altering the age distribution in society (Parse, 1992). The creation of knowledge occurs faster than ever before, causing current knowledge to double every five to eight years and in some fields to double every year (McGuire, 1993).

With these societal changes, competencies essential for nursing practice have changed. Not only will a cadre of basic practitioners need preparation, but advanced nurse practitioners will be needed to meet demands as primary care providers (National League for Nursing, 1993). Critical thinking will be even more essential for nursing practice, promoting greater independence in decision making (Oermann, 1994). Education programs will need to contain a greater orientation to primary care and become more culturally sensitive (American Association of Colleges of Nursing, 1993). Successful programs will convey both intellectual and cultural aspects of health to develop a worldview that values differences (Hegyvary, 1992). Educators must continue to create supportive learning environments for promoting student retention, providing role modeling, and developing effective learning strategies.

Nurse educators must continue to evolve methods that enable students to become life-long learners who think critically and resolve problems creatively. The American Association of Colleges of Nursing (AACN) (1993) suggested that "curricular processes involve the teaching-learning interchange and include such important aspects as role modeling, collaborative problem solving and professional socialization" (p. 7). These ideas are congruent with those of Weinstein and Mayer (1985) who indicate that educating students will encompass teaching them "how to learn, how to remember, how to think, and how to motivate themselves" (p. 315).

1

Several contemporary models suggest an encompassing view for nursing education. This discussion includes a focus on how learning occurs through expert practice, reflection, and experiential learning styles. Research using these models is presented, as well as applications to education and clinical practice. Implications for education and future research concludes the discussion. While these models are not new, they challenge us to view education differently, and to explore the complexity of learning about professional practice as well as the continued growth in practice. Heeding the lessons found in these models will enable nurse educators to more effectively meet practice needs in the coming century.

LITERATURE IDENTIFICATION

To identify relevant literature, searches were conducted using the Medical Literature Analysis and Retrieval System (MEDLINE), Cumulative Index to Nursing and Allied Health Literature (CINAHL), and Educational Resources Information (ERIC) databases. Topics searched included information processing, skill acquisition, reflection, learning styles and strategies, and experiential learning. The scope of the search was subsequently narrowed by focusing on nursing. Additionally, reference lists of selected articles were reviewed for potential sources.

MODELS FOR EDUCATION

Educational models were reviewed and selected on the basis of their application to nursing practice and education. The selected models were ones that potentially provide a direct link between theory-based (classroom) education and clinical practice. Also, each of the models selected are applicable to life-long learning. Three models for education are presented: (1) expert practice, (2) reflection, and (3) experiential learning styles.

Expert Practice

Utilizing the Dreyfus Model for Skill Acquisition, Benner (1982, 1984) identified levels of skilled performance in nursing. Indicating that not all knowledge associated with expertise can be found in theoretical bases or with traditional analytic strategies, Benner suggested that ethnographic and interpretive strategies could identify areas of practical knowledge gained over time and through experience. Using these methods, Benner (1984) reported that development of nursing expertise followed the Dreyfus Model of Skill Acquisition with nurses moving through five levels of proficiency: novice, advanced beginner, competent, proficient, and expert. Each of these phases is marked by unique characteristics.

Novices are those having no experience within the environment in which they are to perform. To facilitate participation in those environments, novices need to be taught noncontextual rules to govern their actions. While these rules provide assistance for gaining experience, they also limit successful performance by failing to guide task prioritization for a given situation. This prioritization occurs only after experience is gained.

Advanced beginners, having some real world experience, begin identifying meaningful aspects or characteristics of a situation learned through prior experience. Aspect recognition permits decision making guided partially by past experiences, enabling nurses to perform at a minimally acceptable level.

Competent nurses, having experience in similar situations for two or three years, begin viewing their actions in relation to long-term patient goals and plans. These nurses more readily identify—through conscious, deliberate, and abstract thought—which actions are most important to the plan and which actions can be delayed or ignored. Because of these thought processes, care becomes more organized and efficient, and glimpses of the overall picture begin to become apparent.

Proficient nurses view situations holistically and have learned from experience what typical characteristics should present in a given context. When deviations occur, such nurses readily recognize which attributes and aspects are important and can modify plans in response to the events. Proficient nurses use maxims or subtle nuances of the situations to guide care and are frequently resource persons to others.

Expert nurses, having moved beyond using analytic principles to guide care, use an intuitive grasp of the situation because of their vast experiential background. Benner and Tanner (1987) indicated that expert nurses utilized Dreyfus' six aspects of intuitive judgment: (1) pattern recognition or the ability to recognize relationships without other prespecifying indicators of a situation; (2) similarity recognition permitting recognition of resemblances, even though they vary from objective features of past experience; (3) common sense understanding representing a deep grasp of culture and language; (4) skilled know-how predicated on embodied intelligence; (5) sense of salience where selected events are recognized as important; and (6) deliberative rationality enabling nurses to holistically view a situation with referents to past situations.

Implications for education. The novice to expert model can provide useful insights for the educational process. Novice learners must be taught principles related to attributes found in clinical settings because they have no experience in understanding and evaluating nursing information (Benner, 1984). Advanced beginners, because of their past experiences, can be taught not only by principles related to fixed attributes, but also by relating principles to situational aspects. Competent nurses, functioning in a manner that is more organized, learn from simulations that allow practice dealing with complex situations. Proficient nurses are beyond the point where context-free learning is effective. They learn best using inductive methods, such as case studies. To further their knowledge of practice, expert nurses need to document areas of performance, comparing, and developing a consensus about patient observations. Benner and Tanner (1987) believe intuition can be taught, but learners must focus on the whole situation rather than trying to break the situation into elemental parts. Viewing expert nurses as they make decisions can accelerate the process of developing pattern recognition.

Benner (1993) offered further suggestions about how clinical expertise might be developed, particularly with students who are already registered nurses. First, experiential learning techniques can be used by analyzing paradigm cases, enabling students to improve skills of reflection on practice and clinical knowledge development. This technique recognizes the importance of clinical practice to education. Students may also benefit from the opportunity to "rework past clinical understandings" through critical reflection on exemplars about past experiences, permitting self-discovery (p. 7). Narrative examination also provides the potential for reevaluation of skills of involvement with patients and families which Benner perceives as critical for moving toward expert practice. Reflection on practice would encourage students to utilize practice knowledge to engage in dialogue permitting scrutiny of theory and its application to practice. Finally, education must empower students and assist them in becoming developers of clinical knowledge.

Clinical application of skill acquisition models.   Benner's model of developing clinical expertise has been applied in several settings. Gorman and Morris (1991) described using an addiction nurse expert, clinical resource nurses, and development of a special interest group to increase practice expertise in nurses caring for patients with addictions. In their experience, novice nurses sometimes used stereotypes and rigid rules to guide care planning for addicted patients causing problematic patient behaviors to escalate. Advanced beginners moved beyond novice practice through participation in case study discussion and mentoring by the addiction nurse expert in direct patient care situations. Advanced beginners became more focused on the assessment of patients on admission and throughout the hospital stay using structured assessment. Because of improved assessment, care plans became more tailored to patient needs. Competent practice was achieved through continued development of expertise by nurses and their influence on other nurses in the hospital. Nurse confidence increased to the degree that they were able to relinquish tight control of patient encounters and consider individual differences among patients. Eventually, some nurses in the interest group achieved proficient practice with some reports of expert practice on the unit. Practice by these nurses influenced the level of practice by other nurses.

Hannah (1993) used Benner's model to establish a competency-based education program for postanesthesia care nurses. She recommended that: (1) case studies from complex care situations be used to facilitate teaching; and (2) an understanding of the characteristics from the five expertise levels be considered when providing educational and clinical experiences required to reach higher levels of expertise. Similar experiences were reported by Whitley (1992) who suggested that expert practice was not accidental and that qualities leading to expert practice could be fostered using mentorship, collaboration, ongoing education, and maintaining practice at the bedside.

Masters, Acquaye, MacRobert, and Schmele (1990) related the shifting role from expert nurse to novice nursing quality assurance coordinator. A particular problem for nurses in this situation is that others still recognize them as experts even though they are functioning in a new role where they are novices. Self-direction was found to be essential and competent preceptors were beneficial for promoting learning. The authors recommended using the Benner model to allow planning of strategies that would permit a smoother transition.

Benner's model of expert nursing practice was applied to a culminating clinical course for RN students with diverse clinical backgrounds and levels of functioning (Carlson, Crawford, & Contrades, 1989). The course consisted of medical-surgical and maternal-child nursing clinicals with a one-hour-per-week seminar. Activities included faculty and student seminars, preparation of a scholarly paper, and clinical experiences. Seminars were context dependent with discussion centering around the limitations of nursing actions guided by context-free rules. A scholarly paper about a critical incident was used to integrate the incident with Benner's domains, current research, and literature. Clinical experiences were opportunities for self-assessment, assessment of other nurses using Benner's domains, and the recording of critical incidents. Evaluation indicated that all activities were successful, particularly writing critical incidents related to clinical experiences. These measures helped to reveal a rich context of student experience that would never have been discovered, using traditional teaching and evaluation methods.

Alberti (1991) described using Benner's framework as a way to level nursing expertise in a neonatal intensive care unit. Competent nurses were often used to preceptor novice and advanced beginner nurses. Proficient nurses, with their development of a specific expertise in neonatal care, were used as care resources and as collaborators with experienced physicians for determining treatment modalities. Expert practitioners functioned as members of the unit leadership team, collaborating with the nurse manager in planning the direction of the neonatal unit. Utilization of the framework meant that nurses had to continually strive to improve practice with expectations for practice increasing as knowledge and skills increase. Alberti viewed implementation of the novice to expert framework as providing motivation for growth and advancing practice. She also indicated that as expertise develops, it must be recognized by new role expectations and titles.

Research using the skills acquisition model. Several research studies used Benner's model of expert practice. Most of these studies focused on increasing expertise in clinical practice rather than expertise gained through formal education. Qualitative research methods were used to describe phenomena associated with skill acquisition. Table 1.1 contains summary information regarding the purpose and findings of these studies.

Two studies presented findings about novice to expert practice development with students in educational settings. Loving (1993) investigated students' perceptions about learning to make clinical judgments. Group and individual interviews revealed that students' motivational orientation and their ability to resolve problems were influenced by their perceptions of the educational context. Based on these findings, Loving developed a model of competence validation describing how students establish their identities as beginning nurses. Loving proposed that education occurs in either an evaluative context, providing extrinsic motivation by external competence validation, or in a learning context promoting internal motivation through intrinsic validation. In evaluative contexts, students believed success was accomplished by getting the right answer rather than experimenting with the possibilities, resulting in cognitive rigidity in problem solving. Students within learning contexts were motivated to acquire appropriate knowledge and skills and became intrinsically motivated by experiences of success in patient-centered care. Validation in a learning context permits students to express what they know and to be open to additional information, leading to greater cognitive flexibility.

McElroy, Greiner, and de Chesnay (1991) used the Dreyfus Model of Skill Acquisition to determine how faculty could provide clinical supervision that promoted skill acquisition, how students learn to make clinical decisions, and the types of knowledge used by students. Master's level psychiatric nursing students were involved in 3 months of

Table 1.1 Nursing Research Related to Expert Practice

Study	Purpose	Findings
Benner (1982) (1984)	Twenty-one pairs of experienced and novice nurses were interviewed regarding patient care situations in order to learn what both had in common about the care. Differentiation characteristics of the two groups were also made for the purpose of learning about how each group described the situation. Additionally, (n = 51) experienced nurse clinicians, (n = 11) graduates, and (n = 5) senior nursing students were interviewed and observed to clarify characteristics of nurse performance at varying levels of skill acquisition.	Evidence confirmed that the Dreyfus Model of Skill Acquisition was applicable to clinical nursing practice. Characteristics of novice, advanced beginner, competent, proficient, and expert nurses were identified. Strategies for successful teaching were offered. Seven domains of nursing practice were identified: the helping role, teaching-coaching, diagnostic and patient monitoring function, effective management of rapidly changing situations, administering and monitoring therapeutic interventions, monitoring and ensuring quality of health care practice, and organizational and work role competencies.
Benner & Tanner (1987)	Expert nurses (n = 21) were interviewed 3 times and observed in practice at least once to identify the nature and role of intuition in expert clinical judgment.	Interviews revealed the 6 aspects of intuitive judgment identified by Dreyfus: pattern recognition, similarity recognition, common sense understanding, skilled know-how, sense of salience, and deliberative rationality. Intuitive judgments were devalued by other nurses, physicians, and the experts.
Benner, Tanner, & Chesla (1992)	Intensive care nurses (n = 105) were studied for the purpose of further explicating the Dreyfus Model of Skill Acquisition. Group interviews were used to gather narrative accounts of practice. A subset of nurses were selected for observation and a detailed personal history.	Four practice levels (advance beginner to expert) were identified. Practitioners at different levels functioned in different clinical worlds, observing and responding to different cues for action. The perceptual grasp of a clinical situation determined the sense of urgency felt by the nurse.

(Continued)

7

Table 1.1 Nursing Research Related to Expert Practice

Study	Purpose	Findings
Corcoran (1986)	Using an information processing approach and a verbal protocol methodology, (n = 6) expert and (n = 5) novice nurses reviewed three case studies for the purpose of comparing initial approaches of experts and novices in task planning, examining the influence of task complexity, and assessing approaches used in each case and quality of plan developed.	Neither experts or novices exhibited differences in initial planning. However, experts used varied approaches depending on complexity of the problem while novices used the same approach. Experts tended to develop better final plans particularly in complex cases. It was concluded that the task itself was a determinant for decision making behavior.
Gordon (1986)	This study used the Dreyfus Model of Skill Acquisition as a framework to analyze job descriptions that formed career ladders. Traditionally, career ladders represent growth of clinical expertise.	The research found that nurses analytical abilities and theoretical knowledge was valued over practical knowledge, experience, and intuition. Career ladders recognized nurses' talking and writing about practice more than their actual practice.
Henry, LeBreck, & Holzemer (1989)	Assigning (n = 60) pediatric nurses to one of three groups, strategies of cognitive processes and performance were used to explore skill acquisition via computer-assisted clinical simulation. Dreyfus' Model of Skill Acquisition as applied by Benner to nursing and information processing models served as theoretical frameworks. Subjects were instructed to either think aloud, to recall decision processes, or given no instructions to verbalize.	Performance on a computer assisted simulation was unaffected by verbalization—i.e., verbalization did not affect clinical decision making, supporting the continued use of verbalizing cognitive processes when examining clinical decision making.
Loving (1993)	Nursing students' perceptions about how they learned clinical judgment were investigated using a grounded theory methodology. Two nursing baccalaureate schools were used with (n = 22) students participating in the study. Data were collected via groups, individual interviews, and investigator clinical observations.	Analysis of interviews revealed that clinical competency can be valued within two contexts, (1) learning and (2) evaluation. These two contexts are interactive through intrinsic and extrinsic motivation. Under the learning context the two elements identified are connecting information and having cognitive flexibility.

McElroy, Greiner, & de Chesnay (1991)	A skill acquisition model was applied to organize observations of graduate psychiatric nursing students as they learned psychotherapy skills. A nurse expert modeled skills and acknowledged the importance of intuition in practice.	It was concluded that becoming a nurse psychotherapist involved a skill acquisition process. Students initially made decisions using a theory based process. It was suggested that other methods to validate knowledge needed to be explored.
Regan-Kubinski (1991)	A grounded theory study with (n = 15) subjects completed 36 interviews to explore judgment processes of psychiatric nurses.	Results revealed present behavior as the most important dimension used in judgment. Categorization based on past experience and knowledge of global patterns also affected judgment. Core categories were discovered to underlie the knowledge base and discriminatory weighting that occurs in judgments. Time constraints, personal feelings, and the setting influenced conclusions.
Steele & Fenton (1988)	Interviews (n =105) and participant observations (n = 50) were completed to examine clinical competencies and skilled performance of clinical nurse specialists (CNS). Benner's domains of skilled performance were used as a conceptual framework.	Skilled performance of the CNS was identified and validated. Documentation of advanced practice can be used as a method for expansion and refinement of clinical practice skills.

participant observation during weekly supervision sessions. Findings indicated that becoming a nurse psychotherapist involved a skill acquisition process. Students made clinical decisions using an analytical, theory-based process, although intuition was acknowledged as being an important part of practice and teaching. The faculty coach identified and worked with students on issues needing resolution. Expert clinical practice was instrumental in modeling and assisting students to identify relevant aspects of situations and perspectives of situations.

From their interviews of 30 clinical nurse specialists (CNS), Steele and Fenton (1988) found that Benner's and Tanner's (1987) domains of skilled performance representing expert practice were demonstrated in the practice of the CNS. The consulting role of the nurse was added to Benner's domains, reflecting a role emphasis of the CNS. Gordon (1986) reviewed the career ladders of nursing units and found that with quantitatively evaluated clinical ladders, analytic reasoning was valued over the intuitive reasoning abilities that are the hallmark of experts. Analytic capacity was rewarded to a greater degree while practical knowledge and experience were devalued. Talking and writing about practice were evaluated more often than actual practice.

Evidence of varying levels of skill acquisition has been demonstrated in both educational and clinical settings. Research by Benner (1984), Benner and Tanner (1987), and Benner, Tanner, and Chesla (1992) confirmed that practice levels of nurses could be differentiated by their characteristics. Support was generated for the concept of intuitive practice. Corcoran (1986) found that expert practitioners varied their approach to care planning, depending of the nature of the task. Domains of skilled performance were identified (Benner & Tanner, 1987) and found to be demonstrated in the practice of clinical nurse specialists (Steele & Fenton, 1988). However, Gordon's (1986) study indicated that intuitive practice was not necessarily valued as evidenced by clinical ladders that rewarded analytic practice.

Reflection

Schon (1983) recognized that traditional education prepared professionals to focus on problem solving where the ends were clear and fixed. He felt this method was contrary to actual practice in which problems are complex situations having confused and conflicting ends. In order to resolve unique problems, professionals are required to exhibit a spontaneous and intuitive performance that reflects a special artistry of practice rather than simply relying on theories from a storehouse of professional knowledge.

Schon (1983, 1987) believed that competent practitioners displayed professional artistry in difficult practice situations. This artistry encompassed three aspects identified as knowing-in-action, reflection-in-action, and reflection-on-action. Knowing-in-action refers to tacit knowledge found in observable everyday performance, instrumental to problem resolution, and yet difficult to explicitly describe. Reflection-in-action occurs when practitioners think about what they are doing and on the knowledge implicit in their action. Reflection-in-action permits critical evaluation, restructuring of thought and influence on further action, and may involve questions such as "What features do I notice when I recognize this thing? What are the criteria by which I make this judgment? What procedures am I enacting when I perform this skill? How am I framing the problem that I am trying to solve?" (Schon, 1983 p. 50). Schon proposed this process as central to the art of dealing with situations of uncertainty. Reflection-on-action follows the completion of the action, and is the process of thinking back about what has been done in order to see how knowing-in-action contributed to the outcome (Schon, 1987).

Schon suggested preparation of practitioners to function in complex and uncertain settings must extend beyond the traditional educational hierarchy, beginning with basic science followed by applied science, followed by the technical skills of day-to-day practice. Rather, education should also focus on the artistry of everyday practice. In order to bridge the gap between knowledge and performance, Schon (1987) proposed a reflective practicum, enabling students to acquire the artistry essential to competent practice. Students would learn by doing, guided by coaches facilitating the processes of listening/telling and demonstrating/imitating. In practicums, guidance is offered to students so they may see the relationships between the means and methods used and the outcomes achieved. Interaction between coaches and students would occur in the form of a dialogue connecting knowing-in-action and knowing-in-practice.

Doll (1993) proposed Schon's envisioning of reflective practice did not extend far enough in terms of the relationship of student and teacher. Doll proposed that the reflective relationship between student and teacher should not be one in which the teacher is recognized as the authority figure, but one in which the student is asked to suspend disbelief in the teacher's authority and to join together in inquiry, reflecting on each member's tacit understandings about the experience. Doll focused on the value of an imaginative realm and inspiration when creating curriculums for professional education. He further suggested setting goals for curricula should not be fixed and precise, but rather allow space for interaction, guiding mutual inquiry on the part of teacher and student. Doll disputed the belief there is a direct transfer of information from the teacher or text to students. Rather, students and teachers must interact to discover the meanings generated through language. He felt education must emphasize interpretation, dialogue, and negotiation.

Doll also proposed that education must no longer be in the central control of the teacher because it fails to encourage the conjoint inquiry that permits meaningful understanding.

Expansion of the knowledge base within the professions as well as the general knowledge explosion led Harris (1993) to build on Schon's concepts by developing a broader expectation of reflective practice. Whereas Schon envisioned reflective practice as encompassing knowing-in-action and reflection-in-action, Harris emphasized the specialized body of knowledge for practice as a complementary source of information for problem resolution that enables multiple sources of knowledge to be utilized for judgments.

Implications for education.   Outcomes of the reflection process between students and coaches are unitary procedures that students grasp holistically. Students learn to resolve problems in a broader way, through juxtaposing and combining other views when established theories do not apply. Learning by doing enables students to develop the ability for continued growth, improving critical thinking, and capturing some of the artistry of professional practice.

According to Schon (1987), the goal of reflective practice is wise action which means applying fundamental knowledge as well as using techniques of reflection-in-action and reflection-on-action. Both aspiring professionals and expert practitioners need opportunities to develop and maintain artistry through forums for developing reflective practice. Practicums for novice practitioners occur in settings similar to real world practice or closely supervised real world practice where students participate in projects permitting them to learn by doing. Dialogues between students and coaches incorporate three aspects: (1) they occur in the context of the students' attempts to practice; (2) actions and words are incorporated; and (3) reflection-in-action is reciprocal on the part of coach and student (Schon, 1987).

Techniques fulfilling the three tasks of coaching include: (1) "follow me" where the novice observes the expert followed by discussion about the action observed; (2) "joint experimentation" where novice and expert engage in joint problem solving followed by mutual reflection-on-action to elicit underlying principles; and (3) "hall of mirrors" where a parallel is created between the interpersonal practice to be learned and the practicum (Schon, 1987). In the "hall of mirrors" technique, novice students and expert supervisors mimic the practitioner to client relationship permitting articulation of a basis for practice. In this student to supervisor relationship, students assume the role of client in relation to the practitioner role assumed by the supervisor. The ladder of reflection where students move up a ladder from activity to reflection or down the ladder from reflection to an activity that makes use of the reflection may also be used.

Finally, guided design is another reflective strategy permitting learners to be given explicit instructions about the decision-making process (Wales, Nardi, & Stager, 1993). Guided design begins with a case study or scenario where student groups read selected information and then answer a series of questions based on the information supplied. Guided one step at a time, students move through decision-making operations followed by teacher evaluation of ideas, feedback about the work done, and suggestions students may want to consider. Printed feedback about what typical student groups might have done is also given, permitting comparison of the current student group to a prototypical group. This combination of student interaction and feedback from the teacher and written materials facilitate reflective thinking on the part of students.

Application to practice. Kataoka-Yahiro and Saylor (1994) proposed that reflection is a significant element in critical thinking and clinical judgment in nursing. Ford and Profetto-McGrath (1994) also conceptualized reflection as an important component in critical thinking. Believing critical-thinking skills must extend beyond problem solving, they developed a model of critical thinking incorporating reflection. Critical reflection was viewed as an essential examination of individual practice and the context so that situational perceptions and individual assumptions guiding practice would be understood.

French and Cross (1992) proposed an educational model shifting from traditional pedagogical approaches where passive students participated in a highly structured course of learning to an andragogical approach where learning sequences were not set and students were permitted to engage in course materials in their own way. Courses would use a practicum approach that initially focuses on knowledge-in-action, and gradually shift to reflection-in-action as student capabilities increase.

Pesut and Herman (1992) used the term *metacognition* to describe the internal dialogue engaged in before, during, and after task performance. Or described in another way, metacognition can be defined as the ability of an individual to think about their own thinking (Pesut, 1990). Pesut and Herman suggested that students who engage in metacognition are more likely to improve their ability to comprehend, understand, and reason. Based on this belief, these authors developed strategies encouraging nursing student utilization of metacognition to enhance diagnostic reasoning and clinical reasoning skills. First students are taught to reflect on interactions from three perspectives: subjective, empathetic or other, and executive control or outside. Then a model explicating the relationship of nursing diagnosis to care planning is introduced, followed by introduction of an Integrated Model of Clinical Reasoning. This model focuses on metacognitive skills including monitoring, analyzing, predicting, planning, evaluating, and revising, which reflect executive cognitive skills. From this perspective, students participate in the process of care planning reflecting on metacognitive questions through the process. The authors believe that use of these models aids student thinking by explicitly identifying characteristics of creative reasoning and relationships among the characteristics that have previously been implicit. Once students recognize these characteristics, their ability to reason is facilitated.

Saylor (1990) conceived of reflection as an integral part of nursing practice and proposed reflection could be incorporated into schools and agencies by having nursing students work together, keep a record of work accomplished, write a journal, and participate in reflective conversations with peers. However, Saylor indicated that for reflection to be successful, time for reflection must be set aside so that rapport can be established with a partner and discussions about relevant practice issues can occur. This time can be built into educational experiences as a part of learning activities. Saylor also proposed that a safe environment, permitting nonjudgmental examination about practice, is essential for the reflection process.

Leino-Kilpi (1990) suggested that if a critical inquiry orientation was expected of practitioners, teacher education would need to include self-reflection. She proposed that once self-reflection is learned, teachers can then apply this technique to analyze teaching strategies. As students learn about the nurse-teacher's role, comparative reflection is used where past ideas about what the job encompasses are compared to the theory and practice of teaching. As the learner moves into the role of the teacher, reflection centers around analysis of feedback from students and content being taught. Reflection permits questioning of principles and promotes discovery of new approaches. In the final stage, reflection encompasses comparing individual ideas about teaching approaches compared to those of others.

Wales and Hageman (1979) applied the concept of guided design to nursing education. Beginning with a situation and a series of questions about the situation, groups of students are asked to come to a consensus about a problem resolution. When the group has achieved a consensus on the answers, the teacher provides feedback to assist in defining the situation. If students have been able to answer the direct questions and anticipate some questions the situation might bring forth, the group is given a continuation of the situation. In the second set of interactions, groups are asked to identify the problem and state the goal followed by teacher feedback. If satisfactory progress is shown, the group is then asked to generate strategies related to the needs of the situation facilitated by group-teacher interaction and feedback. The fourth step is to prepare a plan and take action. As students learn the process, questions become more open ended and the comfort level with reflective knowing and reflective planning increases.

Research on reflection. Only three studies in nursing have examined the concept of reflection. Table 1.2 presents a summary of selected studies about reflection. Powell (1989) studied 8 practicing nurses to discover if nurses use reflection-in-action. Findings indicated that reflection-in-action was present in nurses' descriptions and planning, but only to a limited extent in recognizing value judgments. Powell suggested that prior education has not sufficiently prepared nurses to use reflection. She suggests educators need to consider planning student experiences so the why of care is emphasized in addition to the how and what.

McCaugherty (1991) developed a teaching model to promote reflection and evaluated its use with first-year nursing students. The teaching model was a ward tutorial incorporating small group discussions about the experience of working with a patient for whom the majority of students had cared. Tutorials occurred 3 to 4 times per week, capturing issues in a timely manner. A group receiving classroom and routine clinical instruction was compared to students receiving a similar experience plus the ward tutorials. McCaugherty found students receiving tutorials were better able to provide rationales and exhibited greater depth of understanding for nursing actions than control students.

Sedlak (1992) used logs for traditional and nontraditional nursing students as a method to promote self-reflection about clinical experiences and promote self-directed learning. Logs were analyzed to determine major themes and patterns of learning needs. Clinical logs encouraged self-reflection and facilitated dialogue between faculty and students. Students were empowered by having to direct their own learning and their self-confidence increased.

To summarize, although examples of using reflection in practice were readily available, research on reflection is limited. In educational settings, Sedlak (1992) through the use of learning logs and McCaugherty (1991) through the use of ward tutorials found that students were successful in using reflection as a learning tool. Powell's (1989) study of practicing nurses demonstrated that nurses did use reflection-in-action in describing and planning, but only to a limited extent in recognizing value judgments. For reflection to be most successful, educational experiences should actively prepare students to use reflective techniques that can be transferred to practice.

Experiential Learning Styles

As early as 1938, Dewey recognized the connection between learning and experience. He proposed quality experiences are connected ones, modifying learners in such a way as to influence their perceptions of and responses to future experiences. Dewey felt experiential learning united external situations (the learning environment) with the internal

Table 1.2 Nursing Research Related to Reflection

Study	Purpose	Findings
McCaugherty (1991)	A model to promote student reflection was developed and evaluated qualitatively. The goal of the teaching model was to provide a better link between classroom education and actual practice. Classroom students were compared to ward tutorial students who had reflective questions posed about patients in their care. Data were collected via observations, interviews and diary keeping.	A teaching model was developed that focused on student experiences and also encouraged the development of the teacher's questioning and listening role. The reflective model required a lower teacher/student ratio. The method required active student participation and encouraged thinking and reflecting on events. An outcome of this model was a fuller knowledge of patient care which increased student confidence.
Powell (1989)	This qualitative study examined the use of reflection-in-action occurring in the everyday work of (n = 8) registered nurses.	The reflection-in-action was found to be present in the descriptions and planning, but to a lesser extent in recognition of value judgments and with potential learning opportunities. Reflection-in-action tended to occur more often in community nurses and nurse practitioners.
Sedlak (1992)	This research investigated the learning needs of 1st semester BSN students in the clinical setting. Two groups of students participated in the study. Traditional students (n = 10) were single, less than 21, and recent high school graduates. Another group (n = 10) were above 21 years, married, and included some males. Each student was asked to keep a log of their 10 week clinical experience.	Student logs were analyzed qualitatively. Findings indicated that the nontraditional student saw learning opportunities from the experience sooner and were more focused on self-growth. Traditional students were more focused on the technical aspects of nursing and showed more external motivation factors to their learning. Conclusions indicated that nursing faculty need to incorporate more alternative teaching methods into the traditional nursing curriculum in order to meet the diverse learning needs of students.

capacities (attitudes, desires, and purposes) of learners in a connected stream of experiences that promoted positive growth and movement toward future experiences.

Similarly, Kolb (1984) felt experiential learning encompassed a holistic approach, forming a continuum of adaptive activities beginning with performance and ending with development. He defined learning as a "process whereby knowledge is created through transformation of experience" (p. 38). According to Kolb, the transformation process is continuously created and recreated. Experiences, either concrete or abstract, are grasped through internal reflection or active manipulation and provide a way for individuals to bring out their beliefs and theories, examine and test them, and then integrate them into their belief system. This process permits the opportunity for old, less adequate ideas to be modified or discarded.

Kolb envisioned the learning process as having two opposing modes of grasping experiences (prehension) and two modes of transforming experiences (transformation). Prehension consists of concrete experience abilities where individuals are able to involve themselves in learning experiences, permitting discovery of the uniqueness and complexity of the experience. The opposing mode of prehension is reflective observation where individuals grasp experience through observation and examination from many perspectives, permitting understanding of the problem. One mode of transformation is through abstract conceptualization that relates to the learner's aptitude for using logic to promote integration of observations into theories. The opposing mode of transformation is active experimentation that focuses on the learner's ability to derive practical applications and resolve problems through use of theory. While each mode can be used independently, higher order learning is achieved through combinations of the four modalities.

Four learning styles arise from a combination of the prehension and transformation modalities—convergent, divergent, assimilation, and accommodation. Convergent learning relies on abstract conceptualization and active experimentation permitting problem solving, decision making, and practical application of ideas. Convergers use hypothetical, deductive reasoning that focuses on specific problems. Divergent learners rely on concrete experience and reflective observation to view concrete situations from multiple perspectives in order to generate alternate ideas. Assimilative learners use abstract conceptualization and reflective observation to integrate information and reason inductively, permitting the creation of theoretical models. Accommodators best utilize concrete experience and active experimentation for adaptation to changes through the use of an intuitive problem-solving process.

Kolb (1985) developed the Learning Style Inventory (LSI) to identify the degree to which learners use each of the four learning styles. With this information, learners can see how they have previously processed information. Learning experiences can be adapted to one of four environments and learners can be taught to use selected learning styles to fit that learning environment. In affective learning environments, experiencing the role under study is emphasized, permitting students to reflect on the experience and to engage in discussions of feelings, values, and opinions with teachers and peers. Perceptual environments, focusing on observation and appreciation, assist in identifying relationships among concepts, defining problems for investigation, collecting relevant information, and researching relevant questions. Perceptual environments encourage formation of a personal perspective through the exploration of personal experience, literature, and expert opinion by listening, observing, discussing, writing, and thinking. Symbolic environments utilize abstract conceptualization from information presented through reading, lecture, pictures, and data. Symbolic environments require use of this abstract information for problem solving. Behavioral environments focus on taking action in a situation through applying knowledge to a practical problem of concern.

Kolb (1984) proposed that learning environments may vary to the degree in which they encompass the characteristics mentioned above. Particular types of environments interact with individual learning styles and influence the nature of learning that occurs. Each learning style requires a different type of environment to enhance learning. Learners processing information through concrete experience prefer affective environments, while those who use reflective observation do well in perceptual environments. Symbolic environments best facilitate those who learn through abstract conceptualization, while behavioral environments are preferred by those who learn best through active experimentation. Discussions between learners and facilitators about how learning occurs and the role of the learning environment develop insight about best use of learning strategies to match the environment and matching the environment to students' needs.

Implications for education.   Kolb (1984), Weinstein and Meyer (1991), and Weinstein (1995) consider it important to assist students in identifying their learning style. They proposed that knowledge of learning styles will help students understand the circumstances in which they learn best, either through prehension or transformation. With this information, students can plan strategies that enable better academic performance. Kolb's Learning Style Inventory (1985) indicates the degree individuals use each of the four learning styles. Teachers can also use learning style information to plan teaching strategies for both individual and group needs.

In addition to understanding how to best use their dominant learning style, students can also be taught to recognize situations in which other learning styles would be useful and taught learning strategies promoting success in those instances. Weinstein (1995) indicated that strategy selection increases the learner's problem-solving ability, study skills, content knowledge, and test-taking skills. With learning style information, students become more self-regulated in their learning.

Weinstein (1995) suggested that in order to be successful in learning, students must have sufficient skills, motivation, and a systematic approach to learning. Learning to learn must be embedded in the curricular process. She proposed a process to assist students in managing their own learning. Steps in this process include creating a plan, selecting specific strategies to achieve the goal, implementing the strategies selected, monitoring the progress toward the goal, modifying the plan if needed, and evaluating the plan once completed. These skills are not automatically learned, but must be acquired through guided practice and feedback.

Research on learning styles. Of the models discussed, learning style research has been the most abundant, addressing a number of factors that influence educational preparation of nurses. While learning style research has been conducted for a number of years, previous literature reviews have documented the findings (Merritt, 1989). Therefore, this discussion will focus primarily on recent nursing literature. A summary of recent studies can be found in Table 1.3. Learning styles have been related to academic success, to learning needs and preferences, and the learning environment.

In terms of academic success, Haislett, Hughes, Atkinson, and Williams (1993) found students with diverger or assimilator learning styles had higher grade point averages at the completion of their first semester nursing courses than students with other styles. However, little relationship was discovered between learning style and study habits. Investigators suggested students with accommodator learning styles may need special tutoring or study groups in order to promote academic success in the program.

O'Brien and Wilkinson (1992) studied the correlation of age to learning style and field independence/dependence in learning and the success on the National Council Licensing Examination (NCLEX). They found that, while learning style was not a significant predictor for success, age and field independence/dependence were. Students 36 years of age or older and field independent were found to have higher NCLEX scores than field dependent students of any age. Sedlak (1992) also found that nontraditional students were more successful during the

Table 1.3 Nursing Research Related to Experiential Learning Styles

Study	Purpose	Findings
Bath & Blais (1993)	This study measured the mathematics learning style of nursing students (n = 66). The purpose of the study was to learn if there was a correlation between mathematical ability and the ability to calculate drug dosage.	Descriptive analysis showed that only 10% of the (n = 55) students who solved mathematical problems in a step-by-step method passed the test. Twenty-two percent of the integrated group passed, and all of the global mathematical learners (n = 2) passed. Researchers concluded that there is a correlation between the instrument results used to measure mathematics and the dosage test ($r = 0.41$, $p = 0.0011$).
Burnard & Morrison (1992)	This research explored the perception toward teaching from nursing students (n = 47) and nursing teachers (n = 110).	Descriptive results found that both groups agreed that students should challenge both fellow students and the nursing teachers more. The two groups should also share more information and the teachers should allow the students to release more emotional feelings about their learning process. Teachers wanted students to do more with their learning and students expressed the desire that teachers do more to help them learn. Researchers concluded that more negotiation between students and teachers related to the learning needs of students and the role of both groups in the learning process should occur.

Davis (1993)	This descriptive, exploratory study examined (n = 33) students' evaluation of home visit preparation in relation to personal learning style preference. The Canfield (1988) LSI was used along with the investigator's designed Home Visit Experience Questionnaire.	Although students indicated they preferred highly structured learning situations, their course evaluations indicated they needed direct experiences with a nurse making home visits before making a visit on their own. The experience needed to be very structured in order to complete the assignment independently. Without this type of learning experience the students did not complete the requirements of the course.
Garcia-Otero & Teddlie (1992)	This study focused on the question of whether anesthesia students who know their learning style would have lower anxiety prior to the clinical experience. Students (n = 43) were divided into two groups, a control group who were not given instruction on the meaning of their learning style and an experimental groups that was given instruction on their learning style on three different occasions for one hour.	Using a MANOVA, results indicated that the experimental group had a lower anxiety score than did the control group at the time of clinical experience. Students who knew their learning style and how they processed information had more confidence to begin transferring their knowledge to practice. Also, students whose learning styles matched those of the teacher showed increased learning, which also lowered anxiety at the time of the clinical experience.
Goldrick et al. (1993)	The authors assessed the learning styles and strategies preferences among critical care nurses, operating room nurses, and infection control practitioners. A random sample of (n = 303) nurses responded to survey questions from 108 hospitals in nine geographic regions of the United States.	Findings from the survey indicated the majority of nurses preferred learning strategies that concentrated on organizing information, testing theories and ideas, designing experiments and analyzing quantitative data. The second highest preferred learning strategies were goal setting, creating new ways of thinking and doing, and choosing the best solution to a problem. The learning strategies correlated with the learning styles of the groups.

(Continued)

21

Table 1.3 *(Continued)*

Study	Purpose	Findings
Haislett et al. (1993)	This study examined (n = 100) beginning nursing students' learning style for the purpose of exploring the relationship of learning style to the GPA in the first semester nursing courses, and the relationship of learning style to study skills and attitudes. The Kolb LSI (1985) and the Brown Holzman (1964) Survey of Study Habits and Attitudes were used.	ANOVA followed by post hoc testing (F = 4.57, $p = 0.005$) indicated that students with diverger and assimilator learning styles had higher GPA's. Accommodators had the lowest GPA's. No relationship was found between learning style and study habits. Conclusions were that an assessment of learning style should be done early in all nursing students' academic experience. An introductory nursing course should be offered to enhance abstract conceptualization and reflective observation skills. The accommodators should be offered study groups or tutoring in order for them to become successful in the program.
Laschinger (1992)	This study examined contributions of various nursing learning environments to the development of specific learning competencies, using the Kolb (1984) experiential learning theory. Nursing students (n = 179) at all four levels of a BSN program participated in the study.	Descriptive analysis of the learning style scores indicated that students in the program used concrete, action oriented thinking. Yet, there is need within nursing education for reflective and abstract learning components, especially within the clinical area and the clinical conference. This study suggests nursing education include more reflective learning within both the classroom and clinical area. Including more theory in classes would also be helpful.

| Laschinger & MacMaster (1992) | The researchers examined whether a preceptorship would affect the nursing learning competencies of senior nursing students during their final semester. Two instruments, the Kolb (1981) Adaptive Competency Profile (ACP) and Experimental Profile Quotient (EPQ) were used to measure the pre and post influence of the preceptor with (n = 50) nursing students. | Using a t-test to measure the difference in the mean scores of the two groups, results indicated there was increased difference in planning and leadership scores after the preceptorship than before the preceptorship began. Also, the students showed more reflective skills in theory and experimenting with new ideas. Authors concluded the preceptorship had a significant effect on adaptive development of senior nursing students. The preceptor played an important role in improving the personal adaptation of the new nurse to the profession. |
| Nortridge et al. (1992) | The purpose of this study was to examine relationships between the elements of cognitive mapping results and the academic success at the end of first semester of (n = 325) nursing students over a 3 year period. The Modified Hill was used. | Results of the ex post facto study indicated that 91% of the students were successful. Of the 28 cognitive areas found in the instruments, 7 predictors were computed using multiple regression. These 7 predictors accounted for 13.7% of the variance. Cognitive factors emerging as correlated to predictors of first semester success were: a preference for the use of written materials rather than oral learning along with the ability to sort out information; a high score on independent learning and problem solving; and use of a high level of deductive reasoning. The authors recommended that if student scores on critical variables of cognitive mapping fell below the mean, those students be assisted by faculty role models for critical thinking and problem solving skills in order to be successful in the program. |

(Continued)

Table 1.3 *(Continued)*

Study	Purpose	Findings
O'Brien & Wilkinson (1992)	This study examined the relationship of two cognitive style instruments, Witkin Group Embedded Figures Test and Gregorc Style Delineator scores with age and NLN scores. ADN (n = 72) students participated in the study.	ANOVA demonstrated no significant differences in the main effects or interaction for age and the Gregorc cognitive style scores. There was a significant difference within the Witkin's cognitive styles and age. Overall, students with field independent scores reported higher NCLEX scores. Field independent students, 36 years and over, scored higher than field dependent. Women over 36 scored higher than either field independent or field dependent women under 36 years.
Ostmoe (1984)	This study compared two groups of nursing students in their first nursing course (n = 45) and students completing their last nursing course (n = 47). The two groups were given a questionnaire containing 28 different learning strategies. They were asked to rate their preferred teaching learning strategies using a five-point Likert scale.	The students indicated they preferred the traditional teaching learning strategies, i.e. lecture with visualization and required readings. Enough students indicated they preferred different strategies, especially those in their last semester, that the researcher concluded that students need a variety of learning strategies in order to meet the challenge of the nursing curriculum.
Sherbinski (1994)	This research examined the learning styles of nurse anesthesia students (n = 164) enrolled in 12 programs using the Kolb (1985) LSI.	A statistically significant relationship between learning style and level in an anesthesia program was found. If a student had completed less than 12 months of the program, no dominant learning style was present. However, students who had completed more than 12 months were discovered to have one of two predominantly distributed learning styles: assimilator or converger. Conclusions were that teachers need to be more adaptive in their teaching methods, depending on the level of student.

| Sutcliffe (1993) | Post graduate cardiovascular nurses (n = 30) were given a semi-structured interview on how they learned 5 different nursing topics including: (1) anatomy and physiology, (2) ethics, (3) communication, (4) nursing care, and (5) medical diagnoses and treatment. The results of the interview were analyzed using the preferred learning strategies as outlined by Kolb's (1984) learning styles. | Analysis of the interview data matched the Kolb learning characteristics of the converger and assimilator along with the Witkin's field dependent learning method. Learning via the lecture method was the preferred method for A & P and medical diagnoses. Ethics and communication were seen as needing active extroverted learning, and nursing care was reported to be learned best through case studies. The author concluded that nurses have different learning preferences depending upon the topic. |
| Trigwell & Prosser (1991a) | This study of (n = 122) first year nursing students in a communication course measured the outcomes of nursing students' academic work using both quantitative and qualitative approaches. Four instruments were used to compare the course outcome of the student to: (1) high school grades, (2) course grades, and (3) student questionnaire responses using a qualitative approach for course evaluation, i.e. Approach to Study Inventory (ASI) and (4) students' levels of understanding the course content, i.e., Structure of the Observed Learning Outcome (SOLO) | Results of the study using factor analysis showed that the students' responses to the course as revealed by the qualitative approach played a larger factor in relating to course outcome than did the quantitative measure (SOLO). Students' perceptions of course content proved to be a larger factor in establishing a relationship to the course outcome than did understanding how the students processed the information. |

(Continued)

25

26

Table 1.3 *(Continued)*

Study	Purpose	Findings
Trigwell & Prosser (1991b)	This study investigated the influence of learning context and student approaches to learning on learning outcomes with (n = 55) final year nursing students. Three instruments were used to measure these factors: (1) ASI, (2) course grade, and (3) student written perception of the learning environment over the three year program.	Results obtained using a correlation matrix indicated that the students' perceptions of good teaching related to a deeper approach in the student's study, which resulted in a higher quality learning outcome. A surface approach to learning was correlated with perceptions of a heavy workload, rote earning, and a learning environment lacking encouragement, stimulation, or responsiveness to students.
Yoder (1994)	This study examined the relationship of learning style to the type of preferred computer-assisted interactive video instruction (CAIVI) or linear video. Sophomore nursing fundamentals course students (n = 59) completed the Merritt and Marshall Learning Style Questionnaire (1985) to determine learning style.	A two way ANOVA revealed that learners who used active experimentation learned better with CAIVI. Learners who preferred to learn by reflection or observation learned better with linear video. Further research is needed to substantiate these findings.

first semester of their programs because they were more focused on self-growth and able to recognize clinical learning opportunities earlier than traditional students.

In an ex-post facto study, Nortridge, Mayeux, Anderson, and Bell (1992) used the Modified Hill Cognitive Style Instrument to predict success in a nursing program. Areas positively correlated with success were related to finding meaning in language that is heard, finding meaning in language that is written, preference for independent learning and problem solving, and a preference for deductive thinking.

Bath and Blais (1993) found that a student's learning style in mathematical technique related closely to the success the student experienced with drug dosage tests. Those who used global approaches to problem solving had the most success on tests. Students who used a step-by-step formula process were frequently unsuccessful because they failed to consider other methods for verification of the answer. In order to promote success, investigators recommended that teachers address students' preferred learning styles in ways appropriate to the style.

Several studies specifically examined the relationship of learning styles to specific learning needs or preferences. Yoder (1994) investigated the relationship between learning style and the use of two types of computer-aided learning. She found that active experimenters tended to perform best with computer-assisted interactive video. Reflective learners tended to score higher using linear video for learning. Yoder concluded learning styles do interact with the method of teaching and contribute to differences in learning success.

Davis (1993) examined the relationship of learning styles to learning needs of nursing students preparing to make home visits. Students' preferences indicated they desired highly structured instructional situations. However, their evaluations of teaching strategies indicated they valued direct experience learning situations. In contrast, Goldrick, Gruendemann, and Larson (1993) found that learning style was correlated to the preferred learning strategy of nurses working in critical care, the operating room, and infection control. Nurses in this study had abstract learning styles—either converger or assimilative—and preferred self-directed approaches to learning.

Sherbinski (1994) compared learning style and program level of students in 12 nurse anesthesia master's programs. While students entering the programs showed no dominant style, students completing 12 months of the program were primarily found to have either an assimilator style (40%) or a converger style (38.8%). Garcia-Otero and Teddlie (1992) found anesthesia students who knew their learning style prior to beginning their clinical rotations experienced less anxiety over time. These students also experienced improved clinical performance.

Sutcliffe (1993) investigated whether nurses' preferred learning styles changed according to the nature of the topic area. A convergent, introverted style was adopted for study of anatomy and physiology and medical diagnoses. Divergent, extroverted learning styles valuing active learning methods were chosen for ethics and communication. Sutcliffe concluded that preferred styles varied with subject area.

Four studies examined learning styles in relation to the nursing learning environment. Laschinger (1992) and Laschinger and MacMaster (1992) investigated the relationship of the learning environment to the development of specific learning competencies. Laschinger suggested that nursing learning environments should contribute to divergent and convergent competencies that reflected an orientation toward people and scientifically based practice. She found that clinical nursing courses and a senior preceptorship contributed more significantly to these areas than did other nursing and nonnursing classes. Laschinger suggested that for student nurses to have the highest level of competency in practice, there was a need for more reflection learning, both within the classroom and clinical areas. In their comparison of senior baccalaureate nursing students before and after a preceptorship, Laschinger and MacMaster (1992) found a significant shift in competencies previously considered unimportant by students. Following a preceptorship, students exhibited greater competencies in assimilative and accommodative skills, a contrast from student preference prior to the preceptorship.

Burnard and Morrison (1992) examined the perception toward teaching from the perspective of the nurse educator and the nursing student. They found that while educators thought students should take more responsibility for learning, students wanted teachers to organize and manage learning experiences. Investigators concluded there were differences in priorities regarding the organization of educational experiences for some students and teachers. This preference for traditional teaching methods were similar to findings by Ostmoe (1984). She compared the learning preferences of students beginning their nursing program to those completing the program and found that most students preferred traditional strategies of lecture with visualization.

Studies regarding learning styles have been conducted more often than those about practice expertise and reflection, research problems needing to be overcome include small subject numbers, inconsistently applied instrumentation, and variation of findings. For example, several studies have compared learning style to academic success. Haislett, Hughes, Atkinson, and Williams (1993) found students with divergent and assimilator learning styles experienced greater academic success even though their study habits did not seem to be influenced by their learning style. This study contrasted with one by O'Brien and Wilkinson (1992) which showed that higher NCLEX scores were related to field independence rather than learning style. Nortridge, Mayeux, Anderson, and Bell (1992) found student attributes related to academic success were meaningful in language that is heard or written and a preference for independent, deductive thinking. Bath and Blais (1993) found that students who used global thinking techniques experienced greater success in solving math problems. Based on the different questions raised by these findings, it remains difficult to identify those variables that relate to academic success. This is an area of challenge to nursing education which will need to be addressed.

Several studies identified specific learning needs related to learning styles. Active experimenters learned best with computer-assisted interactive video (Yoder, 1994). Students' stated learning preferences for highly structured learning failed to predict how they valued direct experiences (Davis, 1993). This study contrasted one by Goldrick, Gruendemann, and Larson (1993) who studied specialty nurses and found learning styles of assimilation and convergence to be congruent with the preferred self-directed learning strategies. These two studies can be contrasted to findings by Sutcliffe (1993) indicating learning preferences changed depending on the topical area. Additionally, Laschinger (1992) found that students had difficulty identifying which learning competencies (assimilative and accommodative) might be most helpful in classroom and clinical settings. Following a preceptorship course, students experienced an increase in the assimilative and accommodative skills that were previously felt to be unimportant (Laschinger & MacMaster, 1992).

Therefore, while knowledge of learning styles appears to be useful, coupling use of learning styles with other factors may also be important in determining how to effectively structure educational experiences. It is also important to remember learning styles may be dynamic in that students may shift in their use of particular learning styles depending on course requirements.

DISCUSSION OF MODELS

Nursing is on the brink of the twenty-first century and yet most of our curricula are based on severely prescribed courses of study that do little to facilitate the connection between formal education and practice. Grossman and Hooton (1993) suggested that education and practice need to develop a shared consensus regarding nursing in order to decrease the growing gap between the two entities. This link is more essential than ever before because rapid technological advances demand that nurses continue to emphasize life-long learning. Therefore, nursing education must develop approaches that will not only teach essential concepts, but also teach students how to learn and think. Nurse educators have access to useful models that can be integrated to promote effective life-long education. The models discussed in this paper have complementary aspects regarding the teaching learning process.

The first overlapping area is that of experience. Kolb (1984) and Weinstein and Mayer (1985) identified experience as a critical factor in learning. Kolb was particularly attentive to the nature of the learning environment and of how learning styles influenced an individual's learning in a given environment. Weinstein (1995) indicated that individuals need to be aware of their learning style and strategies enabling them to learn best.

The value of experience is also critical to both expert practice and reflection models, since each requires practice in order to guide learning and future actions. Benner (1984) and Benner and Tanner (1987) documented that nursing expertise is gained through experience, beginning with the need to be taught in codified rules of practice that can be modified as judgment abilities grow through experience. Experience is also an essential component of reflective practicums where learners are offered opportunity to focus on the artistry of practice, guided by coaches (Schon, 1983).

Closely linked to experience is the concept of time. Information must be learned in way that it can be accessed at a later time, permitting integration of new information when needed. Expert practice evolves over time and is coupled with essential experiences that offer opportunities to shift ways in which practitioners think about complex situations. The ability to reflect-in-action and reflect-on-action is a skill that increases over time with experience and practice.

Another common aspect is intuition. Intuitive knowledge described by Benner (1984) has commonalities with Schon's knowing-in-action described as knowing that can not be explained. Benner proposed expert practitioners utilize intuitive actions derived from years of experience. While Benner and Tanner (1987) suggested intuition is representative of expert practice, they also indicated analytic reasoning and intuitive knowledge can work together.

Use of learning strategies is applicable in each of the models. Kolb (1984) believed if learning styles were assessed, then learners could determine which strategies would reinforce their strengths or develop areas of weaker learning abilities. In reflection, strategies to promote reflection included reflective practicums and guided designs. In expert practice, strategies for learning changed with growth of expertise. Context-free strategies where basic principles are memorized could be potentially useful with novice learners to assist in structuring initial learning. However, expert learners, who acquire and use knowledge differently from novices, may find continued use of these techniques suppress expert decision making because formal logic ignores expertise (Benner & Tanner, 1987).

IMPLICATIONS FOR NURSING EDUCATION

As educational models for the twenty-first century are considered, several implications arise for nursing education and research. Learning must be life-long to enable developmental progression from novice to expert. Nursing education can no longer be limited to education within schools of nursing, but must occur in many settings across the professional life span.

To incorporate new strategies into life-long education, the need for change must be recognized by those who teach, both in schools of nursing or clinical practice settings. To meet the needs of a diverse student or practice population, nursing teachers must increase their awareness of options for imparting information essential for growth in clinical practice. As a part of this process, teachers should become aware of their own predominant learning styles and preferences, learn how to use reflective techniques as learning tools, and recognize the skill acquisition level of their learners. Not only will teachers use these techniques for facilitating student reflection, but they will also use them for evaluating approaches to teaching (Leino-Kilpi, 1990).

Nurses must be able to guide their own learning through knowledge about themselves, about tasks, about strategies and tactics, and prior knowledge (Weinstein, 1995). Several strategies can be utilized to accomplish these goals. As students enter formal educational programs, their learning styles will be assessed and this information shared with them. Students will explore ways to develop their strongest learning style, and when and how to use alternate learning styles that will best fit the situation. These strategies will empower nurses to be responsible for their own learning.

Imagine a system of nursing education that spans both formal education and clinical practice. Using Benner's (1984) model of skill acquisition as a framework, the education process would focus on a student's level of skill acquisition. Students would also be taught how professional role skills are acquired and the characteristics of nurses moving from novice to expert practice. While context-free instruction might occur early in the educational process, efforts would be made to provide a context for learning through the analysis of paradigm cases, guided learning, and actual practice experiences. When the depth and breadth of knowledge increases, learning may become more context dependent. As students become practicing nurses, the education process occurring in a work setting would be part of a continuum that started with undergraduate education. The continuum would encompass growth from advanced beginner to competent, proficient, and expert practice as developed through experiences in clinical settings and potentially incorporating continued higher education. This quest to relate clinical practice to education would serve as a point of articulation for schools of nursing and practice settings.

Opportunities for nursing reflection would be a routine part of study in both educational and clinical settings. Questions focusing reflection-in-action and reflection-on-action would be introduced early so students would begin to learn ways to deal with situations of uncertainty. Clinical experiences would serve as a reflective practicum and provide a context for learning. Students would be encouraged to routinely reflect on practice, asking the questions suggested by Schon (1983) regarding the features of the context, the criteria by which judgments are made, the procedures being enacted, and the way the problem is framed. Clinical experiences would be facilitated through guidance and mutual reflection-on-action with experts in practice.

The relationship of students and teachers in all settings would be renegotiated so that students assume a greater portion of responsibility for their own learning. Traditional, authoritarian teaching models would be recognized as nonproductive because learners become passive recipients of knowledge "handed down" by teachers. Doll's (1993) suggestion that the role of future teachers is interactive and guiding would permit space for joint exploration of an emerging reality, encouraging active student responsibility for learning. To facilitate this change in schools of nursing, implementation of process-oriented, rather than content-oriented, nursing curriculums would promote active learning with a more collegial interchange between students and faculty (Meyers, Stolte, Baker, Nishikawa, & Sohier, 1991). In practice settings, this collegial exchange would need to occur between nurses having lesser levels of expertise and those recognized as competent or expert.

In practice settings, nurses would be challenged to build on their expertise. Practicing nurses would take their knowledge of how to learn and how to motivate themselves, and apply it to their practice. Once again, reflection would be a critical element. The process of skill acquisition would be recognized and encouraged by career ladders where intuitive practice is valued over analytical practice. Proficient and expert nurses would be recognized and actively used in clinical practice settings to facilitate growth of less skilled nursing staff. Acquisition of higher levels of skilled practice would be rewarded through increased status and compensation.

While in school, nursing students could develop a portfolio that might contain a variety items. For example, information about the student's learning style preference would assist students and teachers in focusing on ways to best promote success. Part of the portfolio might consist of a record of work accomplished or a journal regarding reflections on experiences (Saylor, 1990). Formative and summative evaluation by both learner and facilitator might also be a component. In order to promote continuity in learning, portions of this portfolio would accompany students throughout their course work, providing evidence of growth in the ability to critically appraise and intervene in complex, reality based situations. The concept of a career portfolio could be extended to practicing nurses. These portfolios could be a strategy promoting reflection-in-action and reflection-on-action and for documenting increasing expertise in nursing practice.

Implementation of these practices would promote life-long learning in nursing education. These approaches are not new, but have yet to be implemented in a comprehensive manner that articulates educational settings with those of practice. Such an approach would permit planning of educational experiences that reflect the complexities of the practice world.

IMPLICATIONS FOR RESEARCH

While literature about expert practice and reflection are found for clinical and educational practice, limited nursing research exists for these areas. Learning style research is more abundant, although research on specific strategies to promote learning is also limited.

Several reasons exist for the popularity of learning style research. One is that learning style research has been made more quantifiable because of the development of instruments to measure learning styles. This contrasts with reflection and expert practice which generally are more measurable using qualitative techniques. Additionally, while it is believed that students learn from their experiences, clinical experience challenges educators (Saylor, 1990). Learning from experience requires accurately remembering what was done and identifying the consequences of actions. Because the clinical world is complex, it can be difficult to achieve this goal.

Research literature about expert practice and reflection tended to focus on practice applications rather than systematic studies. Although valuable, practice application examples lack the rigor of well planned research. Systematic study, both quantitative and qualitative, needs to assess the nature and outcomes of learning strategies and growth in practice.

To accomplish this goal, several implications for research have been identified. First, educational research must be recognized as a valuable means for promoting quality education and advancing nursing expertise. As educational institutions and practice settings endeavor to reduce the gap between formal education and practice, innovative learning strategies must be developed and evaluated.

Qualitative research methods should be recognized for their value in discovering learning and growth of nursing expertise and reflection in practice. Qualitative efforts should not negate the importance of quantitative research, but should offer a method of investigation about areas that do not lend themselves to quantitative study. Studies discovering more about the processes of reflection and expert practice may facilitate codification of practice components that would be useful to novice practitioners.

Studies about learning styles should be rigorously designed with adequate numbers of subjects and sufficient controls. Better methodology in conduct of these studies may aid in reducing conflicting outcomes and enhance generalizability. Learning style research as well as research about other educational models should be carefully evaluated to determine applicability to practice.

Future research might investigate the effectiveness of single learning methodologies as opposed to a combination of teaching methods used in a variety of learning environments found both in education and practice. The concept of reflective practicums needs to be implemented and evaluated for their impact on immediate learning as well as evolving practice. Application of Benner's model of skill acquisition from novice to expert needs to be further evaluated in both practice and clinical settings. Continued documentation of changing nursing student characteristics may also offer insight to guide curriculum development and implementation. Longitudinal studies would offer the opportunity to document evolving expertise in practice, permitting examination of events and strategies that were growth producing.

SUMMARY

As we move toward the twenty-first century, a holistic approach to nursing education and practice must be embraced. Nursing education curricula should integrate current learning methodologies as well as create value for learning as a life-long learning process. Nurse educators and practitioners must maintain an approach that maximizes active learner participation. As models of education are implemented, research about process and outcomes will be essential in promoting sound educational and clinical practices.

Nursing has a rich tradition of meeting challenges brought about through societal change as well as through changes within the profession. Exciting opportunities exist for nurses to craft an educational process that promotes life-long learning so that the profession and the individual can continue to grow as we move into the twenty-first century.

REFERENCES

Alberti, A. (1991). Advancing the scope of practice of primary nurses in the NICU. *Journal of Perinatal Neonatal Nursing, 5*(3), 44–50.

American Association of Colleges of Nursing. (1993). *Nursing education's agenda for the 21st century.* Washington, DC: Author.

Bath, J. B., & Blais, K. (1993). Learning style as a predictor of drug dosage calculation ability. *Nurse Educator, 18*(1), 33–36.

Benner, P. (1982). From novice to expert. *American Journal of Nursing, 82*(3), 402–407.

Benner, P. (1984). *From novice to expert: Excellence and power in clinical nursing practice.* Menlo Park, CA: Addison-Wesley.

Benner, P. (1993). Transforming RN education: Clinical learning and clinical knowledge development. In N. Diekelmann & M. Rather (Eds.), *Transforming RN education: Dialogue and debate* (pp. 3–14). New York: National League for Nursing Press.

Benner, P., & Tanner, C. (1987). Clinical judgment: How expert nurses use intuition. *American Journal of Nursing, 87*(1), 23–31.

Benner, P., Tanner, C., & Chesla, C. (1992). From beginner to expert: Gaining a differentiated clinical world in critical care nursing. *Advances in Nursing Science, 14*(3), 13–28.

Burnard, P., & Morrison, P. (1992). Students' and lecturers' preferred teaching strategies. *International Journal of Nursing Studies, 29*(4), 345–353.

Carlson, L., Crawford, N., & Contrades, S. (1989). Nursing student novice to expert—Benner's research applied to education. *Journal of Nursing Education, 28*(4), 188–190.

Corcoran, S. (1986). Task complexity and nursing expertise as factors in decision-making. *Nursing Research, 35*(2), 107–112.

Davis, J. (1993). Evaluation of novice home visitor preparation strategies. *Journal of Community Health Nursing, 10*(4), 249–258.

Dewey, J. (1938). *Experience and education.* New York: Macmillan.

Doll, W. (1993). *Challenging curriculum icons: A post-modern, post structural pramble.* Atlanta, GA: Southern Council on Collegiate Education for Nursing.

Ford, J. S., & Profetto-McGrath, J. (1994). A model for critical thinking within the context of curriculum as praxis. *Journal of Nursing Education, 33*(8), 341–344.

French, P., & Cross, D. (1992). An interpersonal-epistemological curriculum model for nurse education. *Journal of Advanced Nursing, 17,* 83–89.

Garcia-Otero, M., & Teddlie, C. (1992). The effect of knowledge of learning styles on anxiety and clinical performance of nurse anesthesiology students. *Journal of the American Association of Nurse Anesthetists, 60*(3), 257–260.

Goldrick, B., Gruendemann, B., & Larson, E. (1993). Learning styles and teaching/learning strategy preferences: Implications for educating nurses in critical care, the operating room, and infection control. *Health and Lung, 22*(2), 176–182.

Gordon, D. (1986). Models of clinical expertise in American nursing practice. *Social Science Medicine, 22*(9), 953–961.

Gorman, M., & Morris, A. (1991). Developing clinical expertise in the care of addicted patients in acute care settings. *Journal of Professional Nursing, 7*(4), 246–254.

Grossman, M., & Hooton, M. (1993). The significance of the relationship between a discipline and its practice. *Journal of Advanced Nursing, 18,* 866–872.

Haislett, J., Hughes, R., Atkinson, G., & Williams, C. (1993). Success in baccalaureate programs: A matter of accommodation? *Journal of Nursing Education, 32*(2), 64–70.

Hannah, B. (1993). Establishing clinical competence in postanesthesia care nursing. *Journal of Post Anesthesia Nursing, 8*(3), 187–193.

Harris, I. (1993). New expectations for professional competence. In L. Curry, J. Wergin, & Associates (Eds.), *Educating professionals: Responding to new expectations for competence and accountability* (pp. 17–52). San Francisco: Jossey-Bass.

Hegyvary, S. (1992). From diversity to enrichment. *Journal of Professional Nursing, 8*(5), 261.

Henry, S., LeBreck, D., & Holzemer, W. (1989). The effect of verbalization of cognitive processes on clinical decision-making. *Research in Nursing & Health, 12,* 187–193.

Kataoka-Yahiro, M., & Saylor, C. (1994). A critical thinking model for nursing judgment. *Journal of Nursing Education, 33*(8), 351–356.

Kolb, D. (1984). *Experiential learning theory.* Englewood Cliffs, NJ: Prentice-Hall.

Kolb, D. (1985). *Learning style inventory: User's guide.* Boston: McBer Company.

Laschinger, H. (1992). Impact of nursing learning environments on adaptive competency development in baccalaureate nursing students. *Journal of Professional Nursing, 8*(2), 105–114.

Laschinger, H., & MacMaster, E. (1992). Effect of pregraduate preceptorship experience on development of adaptive competencies of baccalaureate nursing students. *Journal of Nursing Education, 31*(6), 258–264.

Leino-Kilpi, H. (1990). Self-reflection in nursing teacher education. *Journal of Advanced Nursing, 15*, 192–195.

Loving, G. (1993). Competence validation and cognitive flexibility: A theoretical model grounded in nursing education. *Journal of Nursing Education, 32*(9), 415–421.

Masters, F., Acquaye, M., MacRobert, M., & Schmele, J. (1990). Role development: The nursing quality assurance coordinator. *Journal of Nursing Quality Assurance, 4*(2), 51–62.

McCaugherty, D. (1991). The use of a teaching model to promote reflection and the experiential integration of theory and practice in first-year student nurses: An action research study. *Journal of Advanced Nursing, 16*, 534–543.

McElroy, E., Greiner, D., & de Chesnay, M. (1991). Application of the skill acquisition model to the teaching of psychotherapy. *Archives of Psychiatric Nursing, 5*(2), 113–117.

McGuire, C. (1993). Sociocultural changes affecting professions and professionals. In L. Curry, J. Wergin, & Associates (Eds.), *Educating professionals: Responding to new expectations for competence and accountability* (pp. 1–16). San Francisco: Jossey-Bass.

Merritt, S. (1989). Learning styles: Theory and basis for instruction. In W. Holzemer (Ed.), *Review of research in nursing* (pp. 1–31). New York: National League for Nursing Press.

Meyers, S., Stolte, K., Baker, C., Nishikawa, H., & Sohier, R. (1991). A process-driven curriculum in nursing education. *Nursing and Health Care, 12*(9), 460–463.

National League for Nursing Press. (1993). *A vision for nursing education.* New York: Author.

Nortridge, J., Mayeux, V., Anderson, S., & Bell, M. (1992). The use of cognitive style mapping as a predictor for academic success of first-semester diploma nursing students. *Journal of Nursing Education, 31*(8), 352–356.

O'Brien, R., & Wilkinson, M. (1992). Cognitive styles and performance on national council of state boards of nursing licensure examination. *College Student Journal, 26*(2), 156–161.

Oermann, M. (1994). Reforming nursing education for future practice. *Journal of Nursing Education, 33*(5), 215–219.

Ostmoe, P. (1984). Learning style preference and selection of learning strategies: Consideration and implication for nurse educators. *Journal of Nursing Education, 23*(1), 27–30.

Parse, R. (1992). Nursing knowledge for the 21st century: An international commitment. *Nursing Science Quarterly, 5*(1), 8–12.

Pesut, D. (1990). Creative thinking as a self-regulatory metacognitive process—A model for education, training, and further research. *The Journal of Creative Behavior, 24*(2), 105–110.

Pesut, D., & Herman, J. (1992). Metacognitive skills in diagnostic reasoning: Making the implicit explicit. *Nursing Diagnosis, 3*(4), 148–154.

Powell, J. (1989). The reflective practitioner in nursing. *Journal of Advanced Nursing, 14*, 824–832.

Saylor, C. (1990). Reflection and professional education: Art, science, and competency. *Nurse Educator, 15*(2), 8–11.

Schon, D. (1983). *The reflective practitioner: How professionals think in action.* New York: Basic Books.

Schon, D. (1987). *Educating the reflective practitioner.* San Francisco: Jossey-Bass.

Sedlak, C. (1992). Use of clinical logs by beginning nursing students and faculty to identify learning needs. *Journal of Nursing Education, 31*(1), 24–29.

Sherbinski, L. (1994). Learning styles of nurse anesthesia students related to level in a master of science in nursing program. *Journal of the American Association of Nurse Anesthetists, 62*(1), 39–45.

Steele, S., & Fenton, M. (1988). Expert practice of clinical nurse specialists. *Clinical Nurse Specialist, 2*(1), 45–52.

Sutcliffe, L. (1993). An investigation into whether nurses change their learning style according to subject area studied. *Journal of Advanced Nursing, 18*, 647–658.

Trigwell, K., & Prosser, M. (1991a). Relating approaches to study and quality of learning outcomes at the course level. *British Journal of Educational Psychology, 61*(3), 265–275.

Trigwell, K., & Prosser, M. (1991b). Improving the quality of student learning: The influence of learning context and student approaches to learning on learning outcomes. *Higher Education, 22*, 257–266.

Wales, C., Nardi, A., & Stager, R. (1993). Emphasizing critical thinking and problem solving. In L. Curry, J. Wergin, & Associates (Eds.), *Educating professionals: Responding to new expectations for competence and accountability* (pp. 178–211). San Francisco: Jossey-Bass.

Wales, S., & Hageman, V. (1979). Guided design systems approach in nursing education. *Journal of Nursing Education, 18*(3), 38–45.

Weinstein, C. (1995). Broadening our conception of general education: The self-regulated learner. In N. Raisman (Ed.), *Directing general education outcomes.* San Francisco: Jossey-Bass.

Weinstein, C., & Mayer, R. (1985). The teaching of learning strategies. In M. Wittrock (Ed.), *Handbook of research on teaching* (3rd ed.). New York: Macmillan.

Weinstein, C., & Meyer, D. (1991). Cognitive learning strategies and college teaching. *New Directions for Teaching and Learning, 45*, 15–26.

Whitley, M. (1992). Characteristics of the expert oncology nurse. *Oncology Nursing Forum, 19*(8), 1242–1246.

Yoder, M. (1994). Preferred learning style and educational technology: Linear vs. interactive video. *Nursing and Health Care, 15*(3), 128–132.

Chapter Two

ROLE STRAIN, ROLE STRESS, AND ANXIETY IN NURSING FACULTY AND STUDENTS: THEORY AND RESEARCH ANALYSIS

Cecile A. Lengacher PhD, RN

Although relatively few studies have been published related to role strain, role stress, and anxiety of students and faculty, more educators are becoming aware of role demands placed on students and faculty members. Prior to 1988, contributions to the literature and research on role stress and strain were limited (Baj, 1986; Hardy & Conway, 1988; Knapp, 1988; Ward, 1986). The changing dynamics and expectations of higher education along with changes in the health care system have increased awareness of the impact of role strain, role stress, and anxiety on students and faculty.

The language of role theory as identified by Biddle and Thomas (1966) provides a theoretical perspective for this discussion. The evolution and issues related to the concepts of role stress and strain are well described by Knapp (1988) and Ward (1986). Roles may be ascribed or prescribed within society; many aspects of role can lead to competition, unclear roles, or impossible demands. Hardy and Conway (1988) observed that difficult, conflicting, or impossible demands lead to the characteristic condition of role stress. In terms of role stress, role strain, and anxiety, the three major concepts related to competing and ambiguous role demands, several theories provide appropriate frameworks for study: Goode's (1960) theory of role strain; Selye's (1976) theory of stress; and Lazarus's (1966) theory of stress and coping.

Role stress is considered in terms of the social structure; it may be defined as the cause of wear and tear upon the individual and is often in antecedent to role strain. From these external role stressors, role strain which exists within the individual is generated. As viewed by Hardy and Conway (1988), role strain includes subjective feelings of frustration, anxiety, or tension. Role strain is the subjective experience to the wear and tear that individuals experience after role stress occurs.

Anxiety is often a consequence of role strain and role stress. Believed to exist as varying characteristics in both nursing faculty and nursing students, research related to role strain, role stress, and anxiety may provide suggestions for reducing their deleterious effects.

The objectives of this chapter are: first, to critique and review research studies in nursing education that had major variables related to role strain, role stress, and anxiety in students and faculty, and second, to analyze these studies using the Nursing Education Research Analysis Tool (NERAT) adapted from Moody et al. (1988), Nursing Practice Research Analysis Tool (NPRAT). No investigation has examined research in nursing education using this unique approach. This discussion reviews recent research in terms of theory, design, statistical methods, and research findings.

DESCRIPTION OF RESEARCH REVIEWED

The review and analysis were limited to 21 research studies published in refereed journals from 1988 to 1995 that included the major variables of role strain, role stress, and/or anxiety in students who were enrolled in a nursing education program or faculty who taught in a nursing education program leading to a degree. An automated database search using CINAHL and MEDLINE, and a manual search were conducted to identify studies. Published abstracts, dissertations, theses, and proceedings were excluded from this review; only research published in refereed journals was assessed.

Of the 21 studies selected for analysis, 15 (71%) were published between 1991–1993. The largest number of studies were related to role stress, followed by studies of role strain.

The most frequently used research design was correlational 33% (7); 19% (4) were descriptive. Five (25%) of the studies used a quasi-experimental method and only one used an experimental design. Three studies used a qualitative approach and one study used instrument development. Twelve (57%) studies used multisites for data collection. Only four of the studies were found to test concepts and relational statements of the theoretical model. However, 17 (81%) used a nonnursing theory for a framework. Only three studies were funded, two were funded by a local Sigma Theta Tau Chapter, and one was funded by the Association of Registered Nurses of New Foundland.

FOCUS OF RESEARCH STUDIES

The studies were divided into the following categories: role stress of faculty, role strain of faculty, students' stress, role strain of students, and anxiety in students. Of the 21 studies, 11 (52%) were related to stress of students or faculty, 7 (33%) were related to role strain of students or faculty and 3 (14%) were related to anxiety of students. Twelve (57%) studies involved students, and nine involved faculty.

Role Stress of Faculty

Faculty stress appeared to be a major concern for researchers. In a predictive correlational study, Langemo (1990) examined work stress of female nurse educators whose schools were randomly chosen from NLN public accredited schools of nursing ($n = 287$). Stress was measured by the Maslach Burnout Inventory-Form Ed (Maslach & Jackson, 1986), hardiness was examined by the Hardiness of Personality Inventory (Kobasa, Maddi, & Kahn, 1982), and the Blair Exercise Activity Index (Blair et al., 1985) provided estimates of physical activity. Results showed that educators with higher hardiness scores reported less emotional exhaustion and depersonalization and more personal accomplishment. Greater hardiness was associated with lower work stress. The five individual variables that best predicted levels of stress were hardiness, age, education, years in nursing education, and exercise. Five organizational variables that best predicted stress were (1) student contact hours for part-time faculty; (2) task complexity; (3) economic environment of school; (4) number of full-time faculty; and (5) percentage of tenured faculty. Administrators who were supportive, available, and realistic could serve to allay work-related stress. The large sample size produced findings that contributed to the validity of the study. This study was significant in that it tested a predictive model.

In a correlational study, Lambert and Lambert (1993) found that role stress in nurse educators was inversely related to psychological hardiness ($n = 871$). There were no significant differences in stress and hardiness between faculty engaged in faculty practice compared to those who were not. The Role Conflict and Role Ambiguity Scale (Rizzo, House, & Lirtzman, 1970) was used to assess role stress, and the Personal Views Survey (Kobasa, 1985) was used to assess psychological hardiness. This study supported the previous study results, that is, faculty with lower hardiness scores scored higher in their perceptions of stress than faculty who had higher scores. The best predictor of role stress in nurse educators overall was the belief of lack of control in their lives, and that a small percentage of work time was devoted to teaching students. No significant differences in perception of stress were found between educators engaged in faculty practice compared to those who were not. This study provided support to Steele's (1991) study which found no differences in role strain between practicing and nonpracticing faculty.

Goldenberg and Waddell (1990) examined occupational stress and coping strategies of baccalaureate nursing faculty ($n = 70$). Perceived stressors were heavy workloads (clinical and classroom teaching); retaining failing students; failing clinically unsatisfactory students; meeting research requirements; and providing clinical instruction. When the State Trait Anxiety Inventory (STAI) (Spielberger et al., 1983) was used to assess anxiety, a stress-coping scale was developed. The most effective coping strategy chosen for the highest ranked stressor of heavy workload was to seek support from faculty and administrators. Coping strategies for meeting the stressor of research requirements were upgrading research skills; joining in collaborative research; and setting short- and long-term goals. Lack of reported reliability and validity data on the coping-stress scale and the small sample size were the major limitations of this study.

Hunter and Houghton (1993) examined stress in nurse tutors across five colleges of nursing in Northern Ireland ($n = 95$). In their descriptive study, occupational stress was assessed with the Maslach Burnout Inventory (Maslach & Jackson, 1981) and personal mental health, (used to detect indicators of ill health and in studies of stress in the caring professions) was assessed with the General Health Questionnaire (Goldberg, 1978). Results showed that 87% of the nurse tutors were found to be experiencing emotional exhaustion at a moderate or high frequency; 13% experienced low frequency of emotional exhaustion; 98% failed to gain a sense of competence in their work; 53% reported their job to a source of unacceptable stress; and 63% did not feel adequately trained in their job. In response to Mental Health, 70% revealed shared feelings of psychological illness. As in previous studies with American nursing faculty, administrators were found to be needed to listen to faculty. Stress management should be a concern of staff development.

Stressful and satisfying experiences were assessed in a qualitative study of first-time federal grantees by Jacobson and O'Brien (1992) ($n = 34$). Satisfying experiences identified were personal and social rewards (feelings of accomplishment, increased self-esteem, and social gain); material and career rewards (salary, space, travel, equipment, research staff, and enhanced visibility); positive impact on the school of Nursing and the University (respect from faculty, colleagues, and students); and positive impact of research on clinical agencies. Stressful experiences identified were budget; hiring and supervising personnel; equipment and supply needs; access to subjects; fatigue and emotional distress; inadequate and peer support; and timing of needed grant reports. It was concluded that anticipatory guidance needs to be provided to first-time federal grantees, and that administrators and colleagues need to be educated on the various activities of the grant requirements.

Role Stress and Strain of Faculty

One study examined both role stress and strain of faculty. The purpose of the qualitative study completed by Lott, Anderson, and Kenner (1993) was to determine if role stress and strain are present in nondoctorally prepared undergraduate faculty in a school of nursing with a doctoral program. Faculty were interviewed using an open-ended interview approach ($n = 11$). Stressors identified were the inability to meet new role requirements of having a doctoral degree, the stress of too many clinical rotations, negative interaction between graduate and undergraduate faculty, and the cost of a doctoral program which detracted from the undergraduate program faculty support. The most frequent types of role strain identified were (1) the expectation of fulfilling too many roles; (2) followed by not having enough time to fulfill their teaching research and service roles; and (3) feeling pulled in too many directions. Faculty reported the following psychological and physical symptoms resulting from role stress and strain: frustration, anger at the system, inappropriate emotional response, anxiety, forgetfulness, guilt, failure, insecurity, tension, fatigue, sleep disturbances, weight changes, crying spells, hypertension, and headaches.

As recommended by Goldenberg and Waddell (1990), signs and symptoms of role overload in faculty need to be assessed. Mentoring and a support system need to be developed for faculty during the faculty's pursuit of the doctorate. The use of theory as the organizing framework for research questions in this qualitative study could be used for other studies.

Role Strain of Faculty

Three studies examined role strain of faculty. Steele (1991) investigated the opinions and beliefs of faculty ($n = 292$) and deans ($n = 53$) regarding practice of faculty and perceptions of role and role strain. Instruments used were the Faculty Perception of Practice Questionnaire (Parascenzo, 1983) which measured perception of practice and adaption of O'Shea's (1980) questionnaire which measured role strain. There were no significant differences in role strain between nonpracticing faculty and practicing faculty; however, nonpracticing faculty reported having higher role strain. Practicing faculty ranked practice higher in importance in their academic role functions: teaching, practice, research, and service. Nonpracticing faculty ranked their academic role functions as teaching, research, service, then practice. The issue of perception of importance of faculty practice could have great implications for faculty role strain and role stress. The majority of the faculty were nondoctorally prepared and results may have been different if they were doctorally prepared.

Mobily (1991) studied the degree; sources of role strain; and relationship between socialization experiences, personal characteristics, and role strain in tenure track nurse faculty in research universities ($n = 102$). Role strain and socialization experiences were assessed by a questionnaire developed by the investigator. The major sources of role strain identified were role overload followed by role conflict. In analysis of socialization and personal experiences, higher role strain was experienced when the faculty member held a master's degree as the highest degree; taught in the undergraduate program; had clinical and/or clinical and classroom responsibilities; spent ten hours or more per week in clinical instruction; did not have the opportunity to attend faculty development in research: had a difference in role expectations between teaching, research, and service compared to the dean's expectation; and were enrolled in a doctoral program, married, and had children. Clear role demands should be identified if one is going to earn a doctorate while having teaching responsibilities. This study reinforced previous works of Goldenberg and Waddell (1990), and Lott, Anderson, & Kenner (1993) who reported that the recognition of symptoms of role strain was very important. Dysfunctional levels of stress could be prevented through implementation of coping and stress management techniques for faculty.

Factors contributing to role strain in clinical faculty were examined by Piscopo (1994) in a correlational study of faculty and nurse managers on respective units ($n = 31$). Organizational climate was assessed by the Organizational Climate Questionnaire (Litwin & Stringer, 1968), Communication Within Organizations Questionnaire (Roberts & O'Reilly, 1974), and Role Strain Questionnaire (O'Shea, 1982). Significant positive correlations were found between perceptions of organizational, communication, and reported role strain in clinical nursing faculty. Clinical nurse faculty reported less role strain when perceptions of organizational climate were positive, and when perceptions of communication were positive. Orientation programs for faculty were identified to reduce role strain. Maintaining stability of faculty by placing them in one clinical agency may diminish faculty role strain. The small sample size in this study was a major limitation.

Summary.   This review of research on role stress and role strain of faculty supports the need for further investigation of the factors that are related to role stress and strain of faculty and also examination of interventions that could decrease role stress and role strain. Langemo (1990) found that hardiness and organizational factors were predictors of stress. Steele's (1991) study on faculty practice and role strain and

Lambert and Lambert's study on role stress (1993), concurred, in that no significant differences were found in role strain between faculty who practiced and those who did not. Goldenberg and Waddell (1990) found that the highest stressor of faculty was heavy workload and faculty coped by seeking support from other faculty and administrators. Hunter and Houghton's (1993) study on faculty stress, supported Goldenberg and Waddell in that they identified that administrators need to listen to faculty and stress management skills need to be implemented. This was similar to the findings of Jacobson and O'Brien (1992) who identified that the stress experiences associated with being a first-time federal grantee were inadequate peer and administrative support. Lott, Anderson, and Kenner (1993) found specific psychological symptoms were related to stress and strain and their work supported Goldenberg and Waddell (1990) and Mobily (1991) in that signs and symptoms of stress and strain need to be identified.

While factors, signs, and symptoms related to role stress and strain have been identified in faculty, the effects of this stress and strain have not been reported and programs to manage stress and strain have not been implemented. Prevention programs for stress and strain should be implemented. Researchers consistently identify that there is a need for administrative and peer support to assist with stress and strain. Future research should examine and test successful organizational, administrative, and faculty implementation strategies to decrease this stress.

Role Stress of Students

Five of the studies examined stress in students. Three of the studies sampled generic students, one study sampled registered nurse students, and one study sampled both generic and registered nurse students. Burns and Egan (1994) studied the stressful event of the mid-term examination using the Lazarus transactional stress model ($n = 50$). The major purpose of the study was to test the cognitive appraisal component of the Lazarus transactional stress model. Instruments used in this study were the Examination Appraisal Factor (EAF), Personal Stakes Scale (Folkman & Lazarus, 1985), and the Self-Inventory of Situational Response (SISR) developed by the investigators, and the State Anxiety Inventory (Spielberger, 1983). Results showed that threat and challenge perceptions were the only variables that changed as the situation evolved. The best predictor of threat and challenge was control, and the only variable that correlated with grade was harm. Findings showed that the student's ability to manage the testing situation influenced the amount of stress experienced. Opportunities for faculty to increase the amount of control the student has over the examination, such as giving the student experiences with similar questions prior to the examination, would reduce stress (threat) of the experience. This study is to be commended on the attempt to test a component of Lazarus's model in research.

Pagana (1988) also used Lazarus's theory of cognitive appraisal of stress to examine aspects of the clinical experience considered by students as challenging or threatening ($n = 262$). The Clinical Stress Questionnaire was designed to assess the threatening and challenging aspects of the clinical experience. Major themes identified by students were: the threat of feelings of personal inadequacy, threat of making errors and harming a patient, threat of uncertainty or fear of the unknown, threat of the clinical instructor, threat of feeling scared or frightened, and threat of failing. Implications from this study for understanding the student's perspective should assist the clinical instructor to implement strategies to assist the transition into and completion of the clinical experience. It is evident that the instructor should provide the student with the opportunity to discuss emotional reactions to the clinical experience.

In a correlational study, Beck and Srivastava (1991) investigated the perception of level and sources of stress in baccalaureate students ($n = 94$). The General Health Questionnaire (Goldberg, 1972) assessed general levels of distress and minor psychiatric disorders. The Stress Inventory which was a combination of the Stress Incident Record (Firth, 1986) and Stress Scales (Firth, 1986; Frances & Naftel, 1983) was used to assess stress. Results showed that generic students had higher levels of stress than RN students. The prevalence of psychiatric symptoms in baccalaureate students was higher than the general population. This could suggest that these students are at risk for psychiatric illnesses. Improvement in faculty-student relationships could assist with decreasing tension and stress. Major limitations of the study were the small sample size and the lack of information regarding stress scale reliability and validity.

The effects of a stress management training program on baccalaureate nursing students' stress were investigated in an experimental study by Russler (1991) ($n = 57$). The study design and intervention were based on Lazarus' transactional model of stress and coping (Lazarus, 1966; Lazarus & Launier, 1978). Stress was assessed by the State-Trait Anxiety Inventory, Form Y-1 (Spielberger et al., 1983) and emotions were assessed by the Reported Emotions Survey (Folkman & Lazarus, 1985a). The stress management program represented the transactional model and included Basic Stress Concepts (Lazarus & Folkman, 1984); Guided Relaxation (Davis, Eshelman, & McKay, 1982); Refuting Irrational Beliefs (Ellis, 1974); Stress Inoculation (Meichenbaum, 1985); and Assertiveness Skills (Alberti & Emmons, 1978), coping methods were assessed by the Ways of Coping Questionnaire (Folkman & Lazarus,

1985b), and self-esteem was assessed by the Coopersmith Self-Esteem Inventory (Adult form) (Coopersmith, 1981). Results of a repeated measures ANOVA demonstrated no significant differences between treatment groups across time in trait anxiety, reported emotions, or coping styles. However, all groups demonstrated a within-group change in state anxiety, threat emotions, and challenge emotions over the semester. Although the stress management program did not have a significant effect upon the experimental group, interventions such as this need to be considered and tested in research. This study is to be commended for developing a theoretically based intervention, although the small sample size was a major limitation.

Relationships of burnout to life stress, time commitments, and support of RN students for returning to school were examined in a study by Dick and Anderson (1993) ($n = 54$). The Maslach Burnout Inventory (Maslach & Jackson, 1981) was used to assess burnout, the Schedule of Recent Experiences Scale (Homes & Rahe, 1967) assessed life stress, and support of returning to school was assessed by a scale developed by the investigators. Results showed that there were no significant relationships between burnout and increased life stress of 50 RN students returning to school. However, there were significant relationships between burnout and perceived support for returning to school from colleagues and family members. Burnout decreased as support from colleagues and family members increased. Faculty can encourage increased family and collegial support for students returning to school. Results showed that faculty can support students by working with clinical agencies to facilitate scheduling to meet class demands, encouraging students to seek out new advancement opportunities, and precepting the application of new knowledge in their clinical setting.

Role Strain of Students

Four studies were related to role strain of students. Sherrod (1991) investigated the differences between male ($n = 18$) and female ($n = 18$) baccalaureate students in the reported existence of role strain in the obstetrical area. The Sherrod Role Strain Scale developed by the investigator assessed role strain of the student. Using a t-test for independent samples, results showed there were significant differences in role strain between male and female students on the total score and on the subscales of conflict, incongruity, and ambiguity. No differences were found on the overload subscale. Implications for nursing educators is that they need to develop more rewarding educational experiences for the male student, by avoiding stereotyping, using anticipatory guidance, and presenting an equitable perspective.

Lengacher (1993a) compared role strain and self-esteem across academic programs among students who attended stress-reducing seminars and those who did not. The sample consisted of 47 traditional ADN students, 17 LPN transition students, and 24 baccalaureate students ($n = 88$). Instruments used in this study were the Lengacher Role Strain Inventory (1993b) and the Coopersmith Self-Esteem Adult Form Inventory (Coopersmith, 1987). Results of this study showed that there was a significant difference in self-esteem between the experimental and control groups of baccalaureate students, but no difference in role strain was found between baccalaureate students who attended the seminars and those in the control group who did not. There were no significant differences in role strain between LPNs who had attended the seminars and the ADN students who did not. However, there was a significant difference between and within LPNs and ADNs in self-esteem. While role strain scores for all groups decreased, scores for LPNs and ADNs were higher than for baccalaureate students. This research is significant in that it tested a meaningful intervention to assist students with anticipated role strain. As identified by Dick & Anderson (1993), support systems need to be introduced by colleges and agencies to assist students with their strain. Further support systems and interventions need to be tested in research to identify if they are successful or not. This study corroborates work by Russler (1991) who developed interventions and tested them in research.

Lengacher (1993c) tested a predictive model for role strain in RN students returning to school ($n = 86$). Personality was assessed by the Comrey Personality Scales (1970), stage of career development was assessed by the Career Concerns Inventory (Super & Thompson, 1981), and role strain was assessed by the Lengacher Role Strain Inventory (1993b). Results showed that personality, stage of career development, and marital status were significantly related to role strain in RN students and were all explanatory variables in a predictive model. Of the personality variables, neuroticism had the strongest correlation to role strain, and marital status had the weakest correlation with role strain. Because of the small sample size, a cross-validation procedure was implemented that affirmed the results of the stepwise regression analysis. Since predictors of role strain have been identified in this research, educators can assess students for having high role potential strain and action strategies could then be developed such as small group support, advising sessions, or as identified by Lengacher (1993a), by conducting stress-reduction seminars.

In an instrument development study, the Lengacher Role Strain Inventory (Lengacher, 1993c) was designed to assess role strain in female students who work, have a family, and are in school. High reliability alpha coefficients were attained for RN completion students (.94 and .95) and for ADN students (.95 and .93). Construct validity was attained with the contrasted groups approach comparing nonnursing female and male community college students with associate degree nursing students. Reliable and valid inventories need to be developed to measure role stress and role strain in nursing students to improve teaching and promote further research in nursing education.

Anxiety in Students

Three studies examined anxiety in nursing students. Kleehammer, Hart, and Fogel-Keck (1990) examined potentially anxiety-producing clinical experiences of baccalaureate students ($n = 92$). The Clinical Experience Assessment Form designed by the investigators assessed students' perceptions of their clinical experience. Results showed that the highest level of anxiety was expressed by students concerned with the initial clinical experience and the fear of making mistakes. Students identified that clinical procedures, hospital equipment, talking with physicians, and being late were anxiety-producing situations along with faculty observation and evaluation. Fear of making mistakes was identified also by Pagana (1988) as being one of the major threats (stressor) to students in the clinical experience. Faculty need to continue to create techniques and teaching methods that decrease anxiety, and to understand what factors increase anxiety for students.

Bell (1991) investigated anxiety in students when learning a complex skill, and the effect of preclinical skill evaluation on student anxiety and performance when that skill was applied in a patient situation for the first time ($n = 30$). The State Trait Anxiety Inventory (Spielberger et al., 1983) was used to assess anxiety in the control and experimental groups. The investigator found that students who were involved in preclinical skill evaluation and teaching experienced less anxiety than those in the control group who viewed a video tape on the procedure. Through the reduction of anxiety, students can become more involved in other aspects of patient care or the clinical experience. Caution should be taken with interpretation of the results of this study, due to the small sample size.

Stephens (1992) studied the effectiveness of audiotaped imagery in reducing anxiety and improving test performance in first-year nursing students. The State Trait Anxiety Inventory (Spielberger et al., 1983) assessed anxiety. Imagery and relaxation were found to be effective interventions for reducing student anxiety in first-year nursing students, compared to those students who were not involved in the intervention. These were effective interventions that could be provided to students on an ongoing basis; however, they should not be seen as the panacea for dealing with all anxiety. From this study, imagery and relaxation appeared to be effective in moderating negative effects of anxiety.

Summary. It can be concluded that there is a need for further investigation regarding the testing of successful strategies to assist students with their role stress, role strain and anxiety. Burns and Egan (1994), in testing a component of Lazarus' transactional stress model, identified that the more control the student had over the examination, the less threat and stress experienced. Pagana (1988) used Lazarus's theory of cognitive appraisal of stress and found specific stresses related to the clinical experience. Strategies implemented by faculty members to assist with the transition into the clinical experience and completion of the experience were recommended for future research and consideration. Beck and Srivastava (1991), who examined the perception level and sources of stress in baccalaureate students, found that the prevalence of psychiatric symptoms for baccalaureate students was higher than in the general population. They support the work of Pagana in that stress reduction strategies need to be implemented to assist students with stress. Russler (1991), using Lazarus' transactional model of stress and coping as a basis for a stress management program for baccalaureate students, found no significant differences among treatment groups. Students with a low self-esteem tended to have higher trait anxiety and state anxiety, threat emotions, and harm emotions. Dick and Anderson (1993) found that there were no significant relationships between life stress and burnout in RN students returning to school. Lengacher (1993a) in a quasi-experimental study found significant differences in self-esteem, but not in role strain, among baccalaureate students. While role strain scores decreased for all groups after the stress-reducing seminars, LPNs and ADNs were found to have higher role strain scores than baccalaureate students. This study supports the study by Dick and Anderson (1993) in that support systems need to be implemented to assist students with stress and strain.

Lengacher (1993c) tested a predictive model for role strain and found that personality, stage of career development, and marital status were predictors of role strain. Lengacher (1993b) developed an instrument to measure role strain in female students with multiple roles; reliable and valid instruments are needed to measure these variables so that further research can be completed in nursing education.

In a study of student anxiety, Kleehammer, Hart, and Fogel-Keck (1990) found similar results to Pagana's (1988) study: fear of making mistakes is one of the major anxiety-producing experiences to students in the initial clinical experience. Bell (1991) found that students who were involved preclinical evaluation experience had less anxiety than those who viewed only a videotape of the procedure. Stephens (1992) reported imagery and relaxation to be effective interventions for reducing anxiety.

There have been descriptive and correlational studies on identifying symptoms and predictors of stress and strain. Some interventions have been tested to assist with stress, strain, and anxiety. More intervention strategies have been identified and tested with students compared to faculty. Researchers consistently recommend that interventions be established; however, few studies have implemented and tested their effects.

ANALYSIS AND SYNTHESIS STRATEGY

Description of the Approach

The 21 selected studies were analyzed for theoretical and research characteristics using the Nursing Education Research Analysis Tool (NERAT) adapted for this analysis. This 51-item tool was adapted from the Nursing Practice Research Analysis Tool (NPRAT) (Moody et al., 1988). Content validity and interrater reliability ranged from .92 to 1.0 for the Nursing Practice Analysis Tool. Each study was analyzed for these characteristics. The 51 items of the NERAT tool are organized into key research characteristics, theoretical design, and characteristics of the research, to facilitate analysis. The key *research characteristics* identified for each article included primary focus of the article, journal data, characteristics of the principal investigator, funding sources, type of program and students, and type of study related to the practice in nursing education. Each study was analyzed using criteria for the *theoretical design* and *characteristics of the research*. The criteria used in the instrument were based on definitions provided by Fawcett and Downs (1986). Theoretical linkage was adapted by Moody et al. (1988) from Silva (1986). Each article was assessed for level of theory and theoretical linkage as defined by the criteria adapted by Moody et al. (1988). For the theoretical design, the specific criteria for theoretical linkage were: (1) None cited; (2) Level 1—theory or model cited (not linked to research); (3) Level 2—minimal linkage, concepts linked to the research questions/hypotheses; (4) Level 3—theory or model used as an organizing framework for data collection instruments; and (5) Level 4—tests concepts and relational statements of a theory/model. The *theoretical design* and *characteristics of the research* included formulation of research (which includes aims, research questions, research hypotheses); theoretical perspective, nursing or nonnursing; theoretical linkage with the research design; level of theory; research/theory relationship; major research purpose; major analytic focus; instruments, and reliability, validity; design; analysis of results, (which included significance of the results, characteristics of the sample, relationship of findings to previous studies, explanation of unexpected findings, discussion of limitations, and overall assessment).

Procedure

After a computer search using CINAHL and MEDLINE and manual search of the literature was completed on the variables identified for minimum inclusion in the analysis, each study was analyzed using the Nursing Education Research Analysis Tool (NERAT). Data from the tool were inputed into the computer and analyzed using the computer program CRUNCH which computed descriptive data analysis and Chi square analysis on specific items. The following is a description of the results related to the data analysis.

Results and Discussion

Research purpose, theoretical design, and focus. All articles were reviewed for formulation of the research problem, identification, or use of conceptual models or theoretical frameworks and theoretical linkage with the research design, level of theory, and relationship of research to theory.

The majority of studies did not give a clear formulation of the research problem. After examination of the articles, 33% (7) provided only a purpose or aims, 24% (5) provided only research questions, 5% (1) provided only research hypotheses, and it was interesting that 10% (2) provided no written identification of purpose, aims, research questions, or hypotheses. Only three studies (14%) provided a purpose or aims and research questions, one study provided research questions and research hypotheses, and one study provided a purpose or aims and research hypotheses.

The research purpose or aims were stated in 33% of the studies, as compared to Moody et al. (1988) where half of the studies provided research purposes or aims. Although 29% provided research questions and hypotheses in this study, Moody et al. found that 30% provided explicit hypotheses, and Brown et al. (1984) found that 33% had explicit hypotheses. The use of research hypotheses may reflect differences by the researcher on when to use them or not and may reflect the level of research.

Theoretical Linkage and Level of Theory revealed that none of the studies used a nursing paradigm/model or theoretical frameworks/theory. The majority or 81% (17) used a nonnursing theory from sociology, psychology, and physiology. The most frequently used theories were Goode (1960) 33% (7), Lazarus (1966) 28% (6), and Selye (1976) 14% (3).

Each article was assessed for theoretical linkage with the research design. The NERAT used the five level scale identified by Moody et al. (1988). Examination of the 21 studies identified that: 24% (5) had no identifiable theoretical linkage with the research design; 24% (5) cited the theory only, but was not linked (Level 1); 10% (2) had some type of linkage with the research design, with concepts related to the research questions (Level 2); 29% (6) used the theory as an organizing framework for data collection instruments (Level 3); and 19% (4) tested concepts and relational statements of the theory/model (Level 4). The investigator completed an analysis using Chi square to identify if there was a positive relationship between the degree of linkage and confirmation of a research hypothesis. Results showed there was a significant positive relationship between the degree of linkage and the confirmation of a research hypothesis, $X^2 = 15.529$, df = 4, $n = 21$, $p = .0037$. Moody et al. (1988) found that 80% of the studies examined built on previous work; in this study, only 47% of the studies were found to be built on previous research. The effects of trends toward brief reviews of the literature may affect the assessment of this area.

Level of theory in each article was assessed for being descriptive, explanatory, predictive/prescriptive or no level identified. The majority of studies fell into the descriptive level, 57% (12), followed by 33% (7) with no level identified, and 10% (2) at the predictive level of theory. The research/theory relationship was assessed for being atheoretical, theory fitting, theory derivation, model confirming, and theory testing. In examination of the relationship of research to theory, 29% (6) studies were atheoretical, 33% (7) were theory fitting, 24% (5) were theory derived, and 19% (4) were model confirming. The investigator examined if there was a significant relationship between degree of linkage (Level 1–4) and studies that suggested theory building. Using Chi square, results showed there was no significant relationship $X^2 = 8.171$, df = 4, $p = .0855$.

Of the 21 studies reviewed, 81% had some type of theoretical perspective identified. None of the studies used a nursing conceptual model. Almost half or 48% of the studies had no theoretical linkage with the research design or cited the theory only. In contrast, 58% of the studies had linkage with the research design, used theory as an organizing framework for data collection instruments, and tested concepts and relational statements of the theory or model. In this study, the most prevalent theories were from psychology, sociology, and physiology. By comparison, 86% of practice research studies did not use a nursing model and 49% used theoretical models from psychology. It appears that in the nursing education research identified in this study, nonnursing theories are primarily described. Most of the nonnursing theories identified came from social psychology, and psychology. Role theory was an important perspective that was prominent in the review of the research. As nursing moves forward to test models in research, role theories in nursing may emerge as middle range theories which may be applicable to research in nursing today. It is very important that nurse researchers in all types of research identify a theoretical perspective. Theorists and researchers must lead the way to use and explain the theory-research link and faculty in graduate programs need to emphasize theory testing and theory building as recommended by Fawcett and Downs (1986). This author agrees with Moody et al. (1988) who identified that the "failure of the majority of authors to explicate the theoretical perspective or theory-research link is a disturbing finding that concerns all who wish to hasten knowledge development" (p. 377).

Major focus of study related to practice in nursing education.
Each study was assessed for the focus of nursing education practice. Results showed that 52% (11) studies focused on the instruction of students in either didactic or clinical instruction. Six (28%) focused on clinical and didactic instruction, 19% (4) focused on only clinical instruction, and 5% (1) focused on didactic instruction. Of the studies related to faculty, 10% (2) were related to faculty practice and role strain, and 5% (1) was related to role strain in clinical nursing faculty.

In addition, 12 studies were related to the study of students, 11 focused on students, and 1 focused on students and curriculum. Of the 9 studies that focused on faculty, 2 studies focused on faculty practice and role stress/strain, and 1 study focused on stress of first time federal grantees, and 6 studies focused on the stress/strain of faculty related to teaching. There were 2 international studies, 1 from Canada, and 1 from Northern Ireland, and both were concerned with nurse-teacher stress.

Instruction of students continues to be the major emphasis with the research on the concepts of stress, role strain, and anxiety in this study. Clinical instruction was a the focus in 37% of the studies. The concern of researchers with the clinical focus may indicate that there is an increased concern with stress, role strain, and anxiety related to clinical practice, because of the changing acuity level in nursing practice. Nine of the studies related to stress, role strain, and anxiety of faculty, six of which focused on stress/role strain related to teaching. This increase in studies could indicate an increased concern for multiple role expectations of faculty in the academic practice environment.

Design and purpose. Each study was assessed for the major research design and major research purpose: experimental, quasi experimental, descriptive, correlational, qualitative, and other. Examination of the predominate designs revealed that 33% (7) of the studies used correlational designs, 19% (4) used descriptive designs, 24% (5) used quasi experimental, 14% (3) used qualitative designs, 5% (1) used true experimental designs, and 5% (1) used other (e.g., instrument development).

Eleven of the studies assessed were descriptive or correlational for a total of 52%. Explanation of this finding that descriptive/correlational research is being implemented may indicate that the research that is being published is by new researchers. This study found 24% using quasi experimental designs, which is much higher than the use of true experimental designs, but it is similar to what Moody et al. (1988) found in practice-based research. An experimental design was found in one study or 5%, similar to what Moody et al. (1988) found, 6%.

In addition, each study was assessed as to its major research purpose, whether the purpose was factor-naming, factor-relating, explanatory, causal hypothesis testing, or other. The most frequent major research purpose was explanatory, 43% (9), followed by 28% (6) using causal hypothesis testing, followed by 14% (3) using factor-naming, 10% (2) using factor-relating, and 5% (1) using instrument reliability and validity determination.

Description of samples. Each study was assessed for characteristics of the sample. Examination of the samples identified that the mean for the sample size was 148.80, the median was 88, and the mode was 92, the range of sample size was 11 to 871. The type of sampling most frequently used was convenience 67% (14), followed by random 14% (3), 14% (3) used purposive, and 5% (1) used systematic. Sixty-seven percent (16) of the studies included both males and females, 14% (3) only included females and 19% (4) did not identify the gender.

The most frequent type of sampling used was nonprobability sampling with the most predominate being convenience sampling in 67% of the studies. Sizes of the samples were small for the multivariate statistics used in the studies.

Characteristics of the 12 studies that included students showed: 3 studies included samples from both associate degree programs and baccalaureate programs; and 9 studies included students from only baccalaureate programs. Characteristics of the 9 studies which included faculty showed that: 3 studies included samples of faculty from baccalaureate programs; 3 studies included baccalaureate and graduate faculty; 1 study included baccalaureate, graduate, and doctoral faculty; 1 study included graduate and doctoral faculty. The study from Ireland did not indicate level of faculty, but it was assumed to be at least baccalaureate, because faculty were from colleges of nursing.

Reliability and validity. Reporting of reliability and validity determination varied among the 21 studies. Nine (43%) of the studies addressed reliability on current data only on one or more of the instruments, and 7 (33%) discussed reliability on past data only. No study discussed reliability on both current data and past data. Reporting of validity was more sparse than the reporting of reliability, 57% (12) did not report any validity, 10% (2) reported validity on the current study only, 33% (7) reported or discussed validity on past data, and no study reported both past and current validity. Reliability and validity data should be more evident in the research articles, which is a need and recommendation for future research.

Description of analyses, statistical results, and findings. The most frequent analysis approach was multivariate statistics 43% (9), followed by bivariate 24% (5), univariate 19% (4), and qualitative 14% (3). Ninety percent of the analytic methods were judged to be appropriate. Significant results were reported in 86% of the studies, and 14% of the studies used nonstatistical data analysis methods (e.g., qualitative research). All studies had clearly written analysis sections, and all of the studies based the interpretation of findings on the reported results.

Each study was assessed for relationship of findings to previous studies, explanation of unexpected findings and discussion of limitations. In the discussion of findings related to previous studies, 86% (18) of the studies were found to have discussed findings of the current study in relation to previous findings. Twenty (95%) of the studies were found to have explained unexpected findings. It was interesting to note that only 57% (12) of the studies discussed limitations.

Overall assessment. Each study was assessed for contribution to knowledge building, 1 study (6%) was judged to be fair, 10 (47%) were judged to be good in that they built upon past knowledge, and 10 (47%) were judged to be excellent in that they built upon past knowledge and added new knowledge.

Sampling problems primarily occurred with inadequate numbers in the samples, and biased sampling procedures. Design problems primarily fell into the area of using a design, an inadequate sample size, or not using appropriate statistics. Assessment of the studies resulted in six studies (29%) not having adequate samples. The design of each study was assessed for a match between the purpose and the design and 90% (19) were found to have an adequate design that matched the stated purpose.

Each study was assessed for how well the study was explained, from the purpose to the results, and conclusions. Only one study was found to report conclusions that were not evident in the results of the data.

Potential for knowledge building and future research. Each study was assessed for potential for additional research, or theory building, potential for replication, and potential for meta-analysis. All of the studies were judged leading to additional research and would merit

58   Cecile A. Lengacher

replication. Each study was also assessed for potential for meta-analysis, and 14% were judged as having the potential for meta-analysis, and 86% were judged as not having the potential for meta-analysis. Research hypotheses were confirmed in 65% of the studies, and 48% generated a hypothesis from the study.

CONCERNS AND RECOMMENDATIONS FOR FUTURE RESEARCH

Concerns primarily relate to research and theoretical perspectives. In review of the studies in this research analysis, there was not an increase in sophisticated research methods, which should be used in future research. Additionally, sample size and selection need to be considered with future studies so that one has the ability to make predictions and accurately explain outcomes identified in the research.

The lack of nursing theoretical models in the reviewed studies identifies that there are not theoretical linkages occurring between nursing theory/conceptual models and research related to role stress, role strain, and anxiety in faculty and students. In addition, there are studies being conducted with no theoretical basis cited (6 studies identified out of the 21). The movement toward more theory-based research linkages, whether it is nursing or non-nursing theory, is highly recommended for future research. Research should look at stress/strain producers or the critical stressful event that is directly related to nurse educators, and student stress/strain. These studies need to be replicated with full-time and part-time faculty and students across all levels of programming, baccalaureate, masters, and doctoral. Often the statistical design did not have sufficient sample size. Longitudinal studies can be conducted of faculty stressors to see if they change over time. Differences in stress and strain could be examined over time with tenure and nontenure earning faculty. Reliability and validity of instruments need to be reported on instruments used and reported on current data within each study. Lack of having this data available has implications for the interpretation of the significance of the results. The reviewed studies have shown that stress/strain/anxiety is highly evident with faculty and students, yet few reliable and tested interventions are identified to reduce faculty and student stress/strain/anxiety. Stress/strain/anxiety reduction techniques can be tested in research so that students and faculty can benefit. Stress/strain/anxiety reduction techniques related to the clinical experiences, need to be examined overtime. Student and faculty comparisons could be tested across various types of academic programs to investigate differences in levels of stress/strain/anxiety in different programs.

Table 2.1 Summary of 21 Studies on Stress, Role Strain, and Anxiety in Students and Family

Investigator	Categories	Major Design	Sample Size	Major Findings
Role Stress of Faculty				
Langemo, D. (1990)	Work stress of faculty	Correlational	287	Lower hardiness scores were related to work stress. Hardiness and exercise activity improve work stress. Predictors of work stress were: more student contact hours; lower task complexity; poor economic status of school; and higher no. of full-time positions.
Goldenberg, D., & Waddell, J. (1990)	Stress and coping of faculty	Descriptive	70	Stressors identified were heavy workload (clinical instruction), retaining failing students, failing clinically unsafe students, meeting research requirements, providing clinical supervision.
Jacobson, S., & O'Brien, M. (1992)	Stress nurse federal grantees	Qualitative	34	Stressful experiences identified were managing the budget, hiring and supervising project personnel, physical fatigue, emotional distress, inadequate administrative and peer support for research. Satisfying experiences were increased self-esteem, material and career rewards.
Hunter, P., & Houghton, D. (1993)	Teacher stress	Descriptive	95	Nurse tutors (Ireland) experienced high levels of emotional exhaustion. Most common work stressors identified were too little time. The most common request to alleviate stress was more support and appreciation for seniors.
Lambert, C., & Lambert, V. (1993)	Role stress of faculty	Correlational	871	Nurse educators' perception of role stress was inversely related to level of psychological hardiness.

(Continued)

Table 2.1 *(Continued)*

Investigator	Categories	Major Design	Sample Size	Major Findings
Role Stress/Strain of Faculty				
Lott, J., Anderson, E., & Kenner, C. (1993)	Role stress/role strain	Qualitative	11	Negative responses to role stress were frustration, depression, guilt, and vegetating. Positive responses were activity, food, hobbies. Physical and psychological symptoms were identified such as sleep disturbances, weight gain. Types of role strain identified were multiple role expectations demands on time and different role relationships.
Role Strain of Faculty				
Steele, R. (1991)	Role strain faculty	Quasi experimental	345	No significant differences were found between practicing and non-practicing faculty in role strain, although non-practicing faculty had a higher role strain. Faculty engaged in practice and those not engaged in practice viewed these roles differently.
Mobily, P. (1991)	Role strain faculty	Descriptive	102	Majority of nursing faculty were found to be experiencing role strain, a substantial number are experiencing moderate to high.
Piscopo, B. (1994)	Role strain of clinical faculty	Correlational	31	Positive correlations were found between perception of organizational climate and reported role strain in clinical nurse faculty, and a positive correlation between communication and reported role strain in clinical nurse faculty.
Role Stress of Students				
Pagana, K. (1988)	Stresses/students	Qualitative	262	Major themes of *threat* identified by students in the clinical experience were personnel inadequacy, fear of making errors, uncertainty, the clinical instructor, being scared or frightened and fear of failure.

Author (Year)	Topic	Design	N	Findings
Beck, D., & Srivastava, R. (1991)	Stress of students	Correlational	94	Baccalaureate nursing students had high levels of stress and prevalence of psychiatric symptoms was higher than found in the general population. Generic students had significantly higher levels of stress compared to R.N. students.
Russler, M. (1991)	Stress management students	Experimental	57	Stress management training had no significant effect on anxiety between experimental and control groups. However, there were decreases within groups in anxiety over time, for both the control and experimental groups.
Dick, M., & Anderson, S. (1993)	Stress/students	Correlational	50	Faculty showed that there were no significant relationships between burnout and increased life events (time for school and work) in RN students. However, there was a significant relationship between burnout and aspects of perceived support from colleagues and family.
Burns, K., & Egon, E. (1994)	Stress/students	Correlational	50	Stress appraisals of threat and challenge prior to the midterm examinations were negatively correlated. Amount of perceived control over the examination influenced the amount of stress experienced.
Role Strain of Students				
Sherrod, R. A. (1991)	Role strain students	Quasi experimental	36	Significant differences in overall role strain were found between male and female students in the obstetrical area and on the subscales of role strain conflict, incongruity, and ambiguity. No differences were evident in role overload.
Lengacher, C. A. (1993a)	Role strain students	Quasi experimental	88	Stress reducing seminars had a significant effect upon self-esteem in LPN transition students. Role strain was decreased for all levels, but not significantly. Upon comparison, role strain was higher for LPNs and ADNs compared to baccalaureate students.

(Continued)

61

Table 2.1 *(Continued)*

Investigator	Categories	Major Design	Sample Size	Major Findings
Lengacher, C. (1993b)	Role strain students	Correlational	86	Findings validate that personality, stage of career development and marital status were all related to role strain and were predictor variables in a predictive model.
Lengacher, C. (1993c)	Role strain students	Instrument design	327	Results showed that a reliable and validated role strain inventory with a coefficient alpha of .93, .94, and .95 was developed. Construct validity was identified through the contracted groups approach.
Student Anxiety				
Kleehammer, K., Hart, A., & Fogel-Keck, J. (1990)	Student anxiety	Descriptive	92	Examination of potentially anxiety-producing clinical experiences showed students expressed highest anxiety for the initial clinical experiences and fear of making mistakes. Juniors were reported to have higher anxiety than seniors.
Bell, M. (1991)	Student anxiety	Quasi experimental	30	Preclinical skill evaluation and teaching was found to be an effective strategy related to reducing anxiety and facilitating transfer of skill learning from laboratory to clinical setting in the experimental group compared to the control group.
Stephens, R. (1992)	Student anxiety	Quasi experimental	159	Effects of audiotaped imagery in reducing anxiety was identified as an effective interaction in first year nursing students.

A continuing concern is the lack of funding for research conducted in nursing education. This is a concern for all researchers who are committed to conduct research in nursing education.

REFERENCES

Alberti, R., & Emmons, M. (1978). *Your perfect right: A guide to assertive behavior.* San Luis Obispo, CA: Impact Publishers.

Baj, P. (1986). Stress of the returning R.N. student. In W. Holzemer (Ed.), *Review of research in nursing education, Volume I* (pp. 107–124). New York: National League for Nursing Press.

Beck, D. L., & Srivastava, R. (1991). Perceived level and sources of stress in baccalaureate nursing students. *Journal of Nursing Education, 30*(3), 127–133.

Bell, M. L. (1991). Learning a complex nursing skill: Student anxiety and the effect of preclinical skill evaluation. *Journal of Nursing Education, 30*(5), 222–226.

Biddle, B. J., & Thomas, E. J. (1966). *Role theory: Concepts and research.* New York: Wiley.

Blair, S. N., Haskell, W. L., Ho, P., Paffenbarger, R. S., Vranisan, K. M., Farquhar, J. W., & Wood, P. (1985). Assessment of habitual physical activity by a seven-day recall in a community survey and controlled experiments. *American Journal of Epidemiology, 122*(5), 794–804.

Brown, J. S., Tanner, C. A., & Padrick, K. P. (1984). Nursing's search for scientific knowledge. *Nursing Research, 33,* 26–32.

Burns, K. R., & Egan, E. C. (1994). Description of a stressful encounter: Appraisal, threat, and challenge. *Journal of Nursing Education, 33*(1), 21–28.

Comrey, A. L. (1970). *Manual, Comrey personality scales.* San Diego, CA: Edits Publishers.

Coopersmith, S. (1981). *Manual for Coopersmith self-esteem inventories (CSEI).* Palo Alto, CA: Consulting Psychologists Press.

Coopersmith, S. (1987). *Self-esteem inventory.* Palo Alto, CA: Consulting Psychologist Press.

Davis, M., Eshelman, E., & McKay, M. (1982). *The relaxation and stress reduction workbook (2nd ed.).* Oakland, CA: New Harbinger Publications.

Dick, M., & Anderson, S. (1993). Job burnout in RN-to-BSN students: Relationships to life stress, time commitments, and support for returning to school. *The Journal of Continuing Education in Nursing, 24*(3), 105–109.

Ellis, A. (1974). *Disputing irrational beliefs.* New York: Institute for Rational Living.

Fawcett, J., & Downs, F. (1986). *The relationships of theory and research.* Norwalk, CT: Appleton-Century-Crofts.

Firth, J. (1986). Level and sources of stress in medical students. *British Medical Journal, 292,* 1177–1180.

Folkman, S., & Lazarus, R. S. (1985a). If it changes it must be processed: Study of emotion and coping during three stages of a college examination. *Journal of Personality and Social Psychology, 48,* 150–170.

Folkman, S., & Lazarus, R. (1985b). *Manual for ways of coping (rev.).* Berkeley, CA: Berkeley Stress and Coping Project.

Frances, K. T., & Naftel, D. L. (1983). Perceived sources of stress and coping strategies in allied health students: A model. *Journal of Allied Health, 12,* 262–272.

Goldberg, D. (1978). *Manual of the general health questionnaire.* NFER-Nelson, Windsor.

Goldberg, D. P. (1972). *The detection of psychiatric illness by questionnaire.* London: Oxford University Press.

Goldenberg, D., & Waddell, J. (1990). Occupational stress and coping strategies among female baccalaureate nursing faculty. *Journal of Advanced Nursing, 15,* 531–543.

Goode, W. J. (1960). A theory of role strain. *American Sociological Review, 25,* 488–496.

Hardy, M., & Conway, M. (1988). *Role theory, perspectives for health professionals* (2nd ed.). Norwalk, CT: Appleton & Lange.

Holmes, T. H., & Rahe, R. H. (1967). The social readjustment rating scale. *Journal of Psychosomatic Research, 11,* 213–318.

Hunter, P., & Houghton, D. M. (1993). Nurse teacher stress in Northern Ireland. *Journal of Advanced Nursing, 18,* 1315–1323.

Jacobson, S. F., & O'Brien, M. E. (1992). Satisfying and stressful experiences of first-time federal grantees. *IMAGE: Journal of Nursing Scholarship, 24*(1), 45–49.

Kleehammer, K., Hart, A. L., & Fogel-Keck, J. (1990). Nursing students' perceptions of anxiety-producing situations in the clinical setting. *Journal of Nursing Education, 29*(4), 183–187.

Knapp, T. R. (1988). Stress versus strain: A methodological critique. *Nursing Research, 37*(3), 181–184.

Kobasa, S. (1985). *The personal views survey.* Chicago, IL: The Hardiness Institute.

Kobasa, S. C., Maddi, S. R., & Kahn, S. (1982). Hardiness and health: A prospective study. *Journal of Personality and Social Psychology, 42,* 168–177.

Lambert, C., & Lambert, V. A. (1993). Relationships among faculty practice involvement, perception of role stress, and psychological hardiness of nurse educators. *Journal of Nursing Education, 32*(4), 171–179.

Langemo, D. K. (1990). Impact of work stress on female nurse educators. *IMAGE: Journal of Nursing Scholarship, 22*(3), 159–162.

Lazarus, R. (1966). *Physiological stress and the coping process.* New York: McGraw-Hill.

Lazarus, R., & Folkman, S. (1984). *Stress, appraisal and coping.* New York: Guilford Press.

Lazarus, R., & Launier, F. (1978). Stress-related transactions between person and environment. In L. Pervin & M. Lewis (Eds.), *Perspectives in international psychology* (pp. 287–327). New York: Plenum Publishing.

Lengacher, C. A. (1993a). Comparative analysis of role strain and self-esteem across academic programs. *Nursing Connections, 6*(3), 33–46.

Lengacher, C. A. (1993b). Development and study of an instrument to measure role strain. *Journal of Nursing Education, 32*(2), 71–77.

Lengacher, C. A. (1993c). Development of a predictive model for role strain in registered nurses returning to school. *Journal of Nursing Education, 32*(7), 301–308.

Litwin, G., & Stringer, R. (1968). *Motivation and organizational climate.* Cambridge, MA: Harvard University Press.

Lott, J. W., Anderson, E. R., & Kenner, C. (1993). Role stress and strain among nondoctorally prepared undergraduate faculty in a school of nursing with a doctoral program. *Journal of Professional Nursing, 9*(1), 14–22.

Maslach, C., & Jackson, S. E. (1981). *Maslach burnout inventory.* Palo Alto, CA: Consulting Psychologists Press.

Maslach, C., & Jackson, S. E. (1986). *Maslach BI: Manual.* Palo Alto, CA: Consulting Psychologists Press.

Meichenbaum, D. (1985). *Stress inoculation training.* New York: Pergamon Press.

Mobily, P. (1991). An examination of role strain for university nurse faculty and its relation to socialization experiences and personal characteristics. *Journal of Nursing Education, 30*(2), 73–80.

Moody, L., Wilson, M., Smyth, K., Schwartz, R., Tittle, M., & VanCott, M. L. (1988). Analysis of a decade of nursing practice research: 1977–1988. *Nursing Research, 37*(6), 374–379.

Moustafa, N. G. (1985). Nursing research from 1977 to 1981. *Western Journal of Nursing Research, 7,* 349–356.

O'Shea, H. S. (1982). Role orientation and role strain in clinical nurse faculty in baccalaureate programs. *Nursing Research, 31,* 306–310.

Pagana, K. D. (1988). Stresses and threats reported by baccalaureate students in relation to an initial clinical experience. *Journal of Nursing Education, 27*(9), 418–424.

Parascenzo, L. (1983). Nursing faculty clinical practice: Myth or reality? (Doctoral dissertation, University of Pittsburgh) (University Microfilms No. 8411806).

Piscopo, B. (1994). Organizational climate, communication, and role strain in clinical nursing faculty. *Journal of Professional Nursing, 10*(2), 113–119.

Rizzo, J., House, R., & Lirtzman, S. (1970). Role conflict and ambiguity in complex organizations. *Administrative Science Quarterly, 15,* 150–163.

Roberts, K. H., & O'Reilly, C. A. (1974). Measuring organizational communication. *Journal of Applied Psychology, 59,* 321–326.

Russler, M. F. (1991). Multidimensional stress management in nursing education. *Journal of Nursing Education, 30*(8), 341–346.

Selye, H. (1976). *The stress of life* (Rev ed.). New York: McGraw-Hill Book Company.

Sherrod, R. A. (1991). Obstetetrical role strain for male nursing students. *Western Journal of Nursing Research, 13*(4), 492–502.

Silva, M. (1986). Research testing nursing theory: State of the art. *Advances in Nursing Science, 9,* 1–11.

Spielberger, C., Gorsuch, R., Luschene, P., Vagg, P., & Jacobs, G. (1983). *State-Trait Anxiety Inventory (STAI, Form Y).* Palo Alto, CA: Consulting Psychologists Press.

Spielberger, C. D. (1983). *Manual for the State-Trait Anxiety Inventory.* Palo Alto, CA: Consulting Psychologist Press.

Steele, R. L. (1991). Attitudes about faculty practice, perceptions of role strain. *Journal of Nursing Education, 30*(1), 15–22.

Stephens, R. L. (1992). Imagery: A treatment for nursing student anxiety. *Journal of Nursing Education, 31*(7), 314–320.

Super, D. E., & Thompson, A. (1981). *Notes on the career concerns inventory—Adult form.* New York, NY: Teachers College Press.

Ward, C. R. (1986). The meaning of role strain. *Advances in Nursing Science, 8*(2), 39–49.

Chapter Three

THE SIGNIFICANCE OF STUDENT-FACULTY INTERACTIONS

Judith A. Halstead, DNS, RN

Student and faculty interactions are integral to the educational process. Interactions with faculty enable nursing students to develop a sense of professional identity as well. This review critically examines nursing research literature related to student-faculty interactions and the impact of these interactions on the achievement of educational outcomes. Recommendations for future research are included. Described research findings can be used by nurse educators to develop learning experiences that promote collegial student-faculty interactions and the professional development of students.

The literature review was conducted by searching the Cumulative Index of Nursing and Allied Health Literature (CINAHL) database for articles related to the significance of student-faculty interactions. As articles were reviewed, additional references were obtained through reference citations.

Forty-seven articles, published between 1969–1994, were found that referenced student-faculty interactions in nursing education, with 31 of the articles being research-based. Table 3.1 summarizes the research literature that was included in this review. The chapter was organized around the following content areas: (1) socialization process and student-faculty interactions; (2) concept of power in student-faculty interactions; (3) impact of student-faculty interactions on clinical experiences; (4) significance of student-faculty interactions in the classroom; (5) RN students' expectations of student-faculty interactions; (6) student-faculty interactions in graduate education; and (7) faculty perceptions of student-faculty interactions.

SOCIALIZATION PROCESS AND STUDENT-FACULTY INTERACTIONS

The socialization of students into the nursing profession is heavily influenced by interactions with faculty. Professional socialization has

Table 3.1 Summary of Reviewed Research

Author/Date	Data Analysis Method	Purpose	Findings
Baker & Barlow (1988)	content analysis	to identify factors associated with RN student academic success	essential faculty characteristics included ability to relate to RN students as peers
Beck & Srivastava (1991)	t-tests, correlation, ANOVA	to identify levels & sources of stress in BSN students	61% of the students identified student/faculty interactions as a source of stress
Beeman (1988)	parametric analysis factor analysis	to compare how 12 BSN programs meet the learning needs of RN students	programs for RNs only best met RNs learning needs; faculty support was important
Bergman & Gaitskill (1990)	descriptive analysis	to identify characteristics of effective clinical teachers most important to students/faculty	instructor/student interaction skills were most important; beginning students were most concerned about faculty interactions
Brown, G. D. (1993)	grounded theory	to examine how teachers and students perceive distribution of power in relationships	3 planes of power identified: educational, interpersonal, & learning outcomes
Brown, S. T. (1981)	descriptive analysis	to identify effective clinical teacher characteristics as perceived by faculty and students	students regarded interpersonal relations with faculty as more important than professional competence; faculty reported the reverse
Davidhizar & McBride (1985)	descriptive analysis	to determine how students explain their academic success & failure	instructors were rated as the most important explanation of student success & failure
Dixon & Koerner (1976)	factor analysis	to identify constructs used by students to evaluate effective classroom teaching	two factors, individualized prescriptive approach & systematic theoretical presentation, were identified

Study	Analysis	Purpose	Findings
Flagler, Loper-Powers, & Spitzer (1988)	descriptive statistics factor analysis	to identify clinical teaching behaviors that promoted students' self-confidence	5 faculty behaviors promoted student self-confidence: resource, evaluator, encourager, benevolent presence, promoters of patient care
Garrett, Manuel, & Vincent (1976)	descriptive analysis	to identify stressful student experiences	most stressful clinical experiences were patient care & relationships with instructors
Halstead (1993)	descriptive analysis	to determine the perceived extent of collegiality in faculty-student interaction	faculty reported high perceived levels of collegiality than did students
Jones & Jones (1977)	descriptive analysis	to describe the role conceptions of nursing students	nursing instructors were the most influential role models for students
Kelly (1992)	grounded theory	to identify significant influences on development of students' professional self-concept	faculty were most important influential role model
Kleehammer, Hart, & Keck (1990)	content analysis	to identify anxiety-producing clinical experiences of students	student anxiety was increased by non-supportive faculty
Kushnir (1986)	content analysis	to investigate reactions of students to presence of instructors in learning situations	most experienced reactions were anxiety, fear of failure, stress, loss of confidence
Layton (1969)	content analysis	to determine what faculty attitudes and actions helped or hindered student learning	behaviors most likely to help or hinder student learning were those related to relationships between students & faculty
Lee (1987)	content analysis	to identify stressful clinical & didactic experiences of RN students	stressful clinical & didactic experiences included relations with faculty

(Continued)

Table 3.1 *(Continued)*

Author/Date	Data Analysis Method	Purpose	Findings
Mogan & Knox (1987)	descriptive analysis	to identify characteristics of "best" & "worse" clinical teachers	students identified interpersonal characteristics higher for "best" teachers than did faculty
O'Reilly-Knapp (1994)	descriptive analysis MANOVA	to examine types of social support students desire & obtain from faculty	significant differences in levels of social support desired & obtained by students
Pagana (1988)	content analysis	to describe aspects of clinical experience that were challenging or threatening	26% of students indicated clinical instructor was a threat
Pugh (1988)	descriptive analysis	to determine which teaching behaviors students & faculty believe are most important	students indicated they desired more feedback & empathy from faculty
Rather (1994)	phenomenological study	to investigate the lived experiences of RN students	RN students indicated they lacked power & control in learning experiences
Schaffer & Juarez (1993)	content analysis	to analyze student/faculty interactions within an ethical framework	majority of negative interactions reported were related to perspective of justice
Sherrod et al. (1992)	interviews qualitative	to identify students' perceptions of negative & positive aspects of academic & nonacademic experiences	negative external factors included heavy academic load & faculty inattentiveness
Stephenson (1984)	grounded theory	to identify the expectations that teachers & students have of their interactions	students perceived a formal relationship to exist; faculty perceived it to be informal
Stuebbe (1980)	descriptive statistics	to compare student & faculty views of the role of the instructor	Faculty ranked teacher characteristics highest; students ranked nurse & person characteristics highest

Theis (1988)	content analysis	to identify students' perceptions of unethical teaching behaviors	greatest number of identified unethical behaviors involved violation of respect for students
Williams (1993)	descriptive, correlational factor analysis	to determine concerns of beginning nursing students	one significant factor of concern was "faculty support & guidance"
Wilson (1994)	observation & interviews qualitative	to describe students' experience of learning within clinical practice setting	two major goals of students were to "look good" as a student & nurse; faculty evaluation was viewed as adversarial instead of formative
Windsor (1987)	naturalistic inquiry methodology	to understand students' perceptions of clinical	relationships with faculty, staff important to quality of clinical experience
Wong (1978)	content analysis	to identify student perceptions of teaching behaviors that helped or hindered learning	helpful behaviors included: being respectful, willing to answer questions, sense of humor, supportive; these behaviors were most important to first year students

been defined as the process through which an individual acquires the knowledge and skills of a profession, and a sense of professional identity (Jacox, 1978). It is commonly accepted that professional values are initially acquired through educational experiences (Betz, 1985). However, if professional values are to be effectively assimilated by students during their educational experiences, some careful thought must be given to how this can be accomplished.

The values of a profession are demonstrated through the profession's practitioners who serve as role models (Kramer, 1968). During the educational process, faculty serve as the primary role models for students. Faculty function as socializing agents by teaching and modeling the professional role, and by displaying commitment to the values of the nursing profession (AACN, 1986). Beliefs and attitudes of nursing faculty have a great impact on the developing professional identity of students (Betz, 1985).

Undergraduate nursing students consider faculty to be influential role models, especially early in the educational process (Jones & Jones, 1977; Kelly, 1992). Effective faculty role models consciously and consistently demonstrate desirable behaviors for students. Influential role model behaviors include being supportive, listening to students, exhibiting a sense of humor, and spending the time necessary to do a good job (Kelly, 1992). Collaborative, collegial student-faculty relationships provide an environment that promotes growth opportunities for both parties, professional respect and cohesiveness, and the transferal of other positive professional behaviors and values (Griffith & Bakanauskas, 1983; Hammer & Tufts, 1985).

CONCEPT OF POWER IN
STUDENT-FACULTY INTERACTIONS

While it is obvious that collaborative, collegial relationships between students and faculty are desirable, one must question how often students experience such relationships with faculty. The literature review revealed that the concept of power was an underlying theme throughout most student-faculty interactions. The manner in which students described their relationships with faculty indicates that students are acutely aware of the power that exists within the role of teacher.

Brown (1993) conducted a study to determine how faculty and students perceived the distribution of power in their relationships, and how the balance of power was created and maintained. Using a grounded theory approach, Brown interviewed five students and four nurse educators. Faculty and students agreed that there are essentially three planes of power in the student-teacher relationship. These three planes of power exist within the educational process, interpersonal relationships, and learning outcomes. Students and faculty agreed that faculty have the most control over the educational process by virtue of their *position power*. *Interpersonal power* was perceived by both students and faculty to vary widely from teacher to teacher. Students were more inclined to emphasize the importance of this power plane than faculty and, in fact, considered it more important than the *educational power* held by faculty. However, both groups agreed that students hold the ultimate power over learning outcomes. While faculty may control the educational process, students can choose to learn or not to learn, to listen or not to listen. The student emphasis on the importance of interpersonal relationships should not be dismissed, but rather acknowledged by faculty. Empowerment of students is more likely to occur through collegial faculty relationships that emphasize teacher approachability, mutual respect, and healthy self-disclosure. Study limitations included the small, nonrandomized, convenience sample that precludes generalizability of the findings.

The issue of power in student-faculty relationships was also addressed by Rather (1994) who investigated the experiences of registered nurses who returned to school. Using Heideggerian phenomenology, Rather analyzed the interview responses of fifteen RN students who were enrolled in three different baccalaureate programs. The RN students were asked to describe what it was like to return to school. Analysis of the interviews indicated that the students experienced feeling a lack of power and control in their educational experiences. Students described these feelings as resulting from oppressive teaching strategies that prescribed thoughts, values, and behaviors, and devalued the RN's experience-based knowledge. Rather emphasized that faculty had not deliberately instilled these feelings of oppression, but that these feelings were the unintentional result of faculty teaching practices. Rather suggested that faculty reconsider their teaching strategies and strive to foster learning environments that would empower the RN students to be autonomous equals in the classroom.

An instructor's demand for control and power in the teaching environment can be seriously disruptive for students. Students respond to such situations with a sense of being manipulated and feeling vulnerable (Halldorsdottir, 1990). Such misuse of power in student-faculty interactions has ethical implications. In Theis' (1988) study of nursing students' perceptions of unethical teaching behaviors, 167 senior baccalaureate students described incidents that they perceived to be unethical. The largest number of reported unethical incidents involved violations of respect for students. Faculty behaviors cited as examples of this violation included rudeness, authoritarianism, sarcasm, ridicule, belittling, and insensitivity toward the learner. These behaviors occurred in classroom and clinical settings. The validity of the classification system used in this study was not addressed by Theis.

Schaffer and Juarez (1993) also studied nursing students' perceptions of student-faculty interactions within an ethical framework. Twenty-two students were asked to maintain a journal during their senior year in an effort to explore how their educational experiences impacted their professional development and their self-concept. Analysis of the journal entries revealed that 17 of the students recorded a total of 26 separate descriptions of student-faculty interactions written from an ethical perspective. Of these 26 descriptions, 22 expressed negative viewpoints of student-teacher interactions. The student descriptions primarily reflected a perceived lack of respect for student autonomy, and a lack of justice, beneficence, and caring as evidenced through faculty behaviors. Schaffer and Juarez recommended replication of the study and additional research that would compare faculty and student perspectives of the same interactions. A limitation of this study was that the validity of the categorization of ethical perspectives was not established.

Relationships that are based on issues of power and control cannot be characterized as caring and collegial in nature. The concept of caring and how it is experienced by students through student/faculty interactions has been the focus of numerous phenomenological studies (Appleton, 1990; Beck, 1991; Hughes, 1992; Miller, Haber, & Byrne, 1990; Nelms, 1990). The role modeling of caring behaviors by faculty can help students integrate caring behaviors into their professional interactions with clients and others (Beck, 1991). An extensive review of this literature was conducted by Frank (1994) and is not repeated in this review.

ACHIEVEMENT OF EDUCATIONAL OUTCOMES

The review of the literature indicated that student-faculty interactions have the potential to positively or negatively impact students' clinical performances, classroom performances, and program satisfaction. While the majority of the research emphasizes the importance of collegial student-faculty interactions from the student perspective, it does not indicate how often students actually experience collegiality in these interactions. Most studies have been conducted within undergraduate and RN-degree programs, with little emphasis on graduate students' perspectives.

Impact of Student-Faculty Interactions on Clinical Experiences

The influence of student-faculty interactions on the quality of the student's clinical experience has been well documented. In Windsor's

(1987) study, nine senior nursing students clearly identified that the quality of their clinical learning experiences was affected by their relationships with faculty. Students identified desirable qualities for clinical faculty to be respect, humor, warmth, honesty, and enthusiasm. Students also wanted to be able to ask questions without fear of embarrassment or harassment by the instructor, and to receive frequent, private feedback about their performance. Windsor established trustworthiness for this naturalistic inquiry study through the use of Guba's major criteria of credibility, transferability, dependability, and confirmability. Findings similar to Windsor's were reported by Wong (1978) in her study of 14 diploma nursing students. Students were asked to generate a listing of teacher behaviors that facilitated or hindered learning. Facilitative teacher behaviors included showing respect for students, willingness to answer questions, providing encouragement, displaying a sense of humor, and displaying confidence in students. Hindering behaviors included posing a threat, using sarcasm, emphasizing student mistakes, correcting students in front of others, acting superior, and belittling students. A limitation of this study was the small convenience sample size.

From the review of additional research studies related to the significance of student-faculty interactions in clinical instruction, two major themes could be identified. The first theme was the issue of evaluation versus learning in the clinical setting. Wilson (1994) noted that students developed their perspective of learning in the clinical setting as they interacted with the environment. The 30 senior level baccalaureate students who were interviewed in Wilson's qualitative study viewed interactions with faculty as primarily evaluative in nature, with student learning tending to occur outside the context of their interactions with faculty. These students expressed the need to "look good" to faculty and thus tended to utilize staff to obtain answers to their questions about clinical practice. The majority of students considered evaluation by faculty to be adversarial instead of formative, expressing feelings that they could not make mistakes and must correctly answer all of their instructor's questions. Limitations to Wilson's study included a small, convenience sample of students enrolled in one school of nursing, thus affecting the generalizability of findings.

Flagler, Loper-Powers, and Spitzer (1988), in their study of 139 baccalaureate students, also found that the clinical setting provided an environment from which students received faculty feedback regarding their abilities to be nurses. Such cues from faculty could either positively or negatively influence the student's professional development. Faculty who positively impacted the students' self-confidence and professional development were those faculty whom students considered to be encouragers, resources, and a benevolent presence in the clinical setting. Flagler et al. concluded that focusing on evaluation behaviors alone may impede the professional development of nursing students. Study limitations included use of a nonrandomized sample and not establishing validity and reliability of the questionnaire.

The theme of evaluation also appeared in Kushnir's (1986) qualitative study that investigated the reactions of nursing students to the presence of instructors in learning situations. Students were asked to provide a written description of a stressful interpersonal encounter with a person of higher status. Of the 28 students who participated, 71% identified an incident involving a nursing instructor. The incidents typically occurred when the student was involved in a "first-time" clinical experience and interpreted the instructor's feedback of their performance to be evaluative and critical. The critical feedback resulted in the students experiencing a variety of physiological and psychological reactions with the primary response being one of anxiety, stress, fear of failure, and loss of confidence.

Kushnir's study touched on the second theme to emerge from the review of research related to clinical instruction and student-faculty interactions. The second and predominant theme was that of the stress and anxiety students experienced in clinical learning situations as a result of interactions with faculty. Kleehammer, Hart, and Keck (1990) surveyed a convenience sample of 39 junior and 53 senior nursing students to identify potentially anxiety-producing clinical situations. The most common anxiety-producing situation reported by students was that of negative interactions with faculty, especially when the interactions were related to observation and evaluation of the student.

The fact that students frequently associate stressful clinical events with negative faculty interactions is not new. Garrett, Manuel, and Vincent (1976) and Pagana (1988) conducted separate qualitative studies ($n = 111$; $n = 262$) to identify stressful experiences of undergraduate nursing students. In both studies, students identified their interpersonal relationships with clinical faculty as one of the major stressors present in the clinical setting. While Pagana's study explored the stressors of students in their first clinical experiences, Garrett et al. surveyed students throughout their educational experiences. In this study, Garrett et al. reported that as students progressed through the nursing program, their reported incidents of stressful experiences with faculty decreased. This indicated that student perceptions and expectations of faculty interactions may change as the students' experience level changes. A limitation of both studies was the subjective, self-reporting nature of the studies. And finally, Beck and Srivastava (1991) surveyed 94 Canadian nursing students in one university school of nursing to identify the sources and levels of stress experienced by baccalaureate students. In this study, 61% of the respondents identified the atmosphere created by clinical faculty as a major source of stress. One limitation of this study was that reliability of the stress inventory tool was not established.

It is apparent from these studies that students do not necessarily perceive that they receive the support they desire from clinical faculty. This perceived lack of interpersonal support leads to additional stress in clinical situations that are already fraught with fear and uncertainty. What types of faculty support do students desire during their clinical experiences? In a descriptive cross-sectional designed survey, O'Reilly-Knapp (1994) studied the desired and obtained levels of social support as perceived by 242 junior and senior baccalaureate nursing students. The results ($p < .001$) indicated that students were not receiving the levels of social support that they desired from faculty during clinical experiences. The types of support that students most desired were categorized as directive guidance and nondirective support with juniors desiring significantly ($p < .05$) more directive guidance than the senior students. This again indicates that as students progress through their educational programs the types of supportive interactions they desire with faculty varies. O'Reilly-Knapp identified two limitations to the study: (1) the sample was obtained from only three schools and (2) while the social support tool appeared to have validity and reliability, it was not standardized.

Significance of Student-Faculty Interactions in the Classroom

In comparison to the number of clinical setting studies, very few research studies have been conducted to determine the significance of student-faculty interactions on the success of students in the classroom setting. Layton (1969) conducted one of the earliest studies to determine how instructor attitudes and behaviors affected student learning. She surveyed 141 nursing students who identified student-faculty interactions as the behaviors that most often affected student learning. Faculty who exhibited collegial behaviors such as providing encouragement, showing acceptance of the student, and being willing to answer questions, were considered most helpful in promoting learning. Faculty who displayed noncollegial characteristics, such as "being threatening and sarcastic," "acting superior," "punishing students for lacking knowledge," and "correcting students in front of others," hindered learning. Layton emphasized that faculty are most effective in conveying knowledge to students when they relate to students in a positive manner.

Dixon and Koerner (1976) attempted to identify the constructs students use to determine the classroom effectiveness of faculty. Prior to surveying students, the authors identified six theoretical constructs that they felt were related to effective classroom teaching. These six constructs were: (1) planning and organization, (2) mastery of content, (3) clarity of presentation, (4) levels of thinking, (5) involvement and receptivity, and (6) fairness. Content validity of the six constructs was established by faculty. The tool was distributed to 1,340 students (1,191 undergraduate, 51 graduate, and 53 of unknown classification) who were asked to evaluate the faculty with whom they had contact. All faculty ($n = 39$) within the school were asked to collect anonymous evaluations about their classroom effectiveness. Factor analysis indicated that instead of the anticipated six factors, only two factors emerged to describe effective faculty behaviors in the classroom. The first factor, which accounted for 24.7% of the variance in the student responses, was labeled "individualized prescriptive approach" and included items related to faculty responding to students as individuals. The second factor, which accounted for 24.5% of the total variance, focused on classroom presentation and was labeled "systematic theoretical orientation." One important implication of this study was that student and faculty perceptions of effective classroom teaching may differ. Students were more inclined to value teacher behaviors that demonstrated awareness of the individual student's needs relative to evaluation, feedback, and guidance. A limitation of this study was the small number of faculty who were evaluated. It should also be noted that while only a small number of graduate students were included in the sample, it is reasonable to assume that they may have different perceptions of effective teaching behaviors than undergraduate students.

Davidhizar and McBride (1985) used attribution theory to describe how nursing students explained their feelings of success and failure in the provision of nursing care and the mastery of theory. Attribution theory describes achievement-related behaviors in terms of good or bad luck, ability, ease of task, or effort. Locus of control may be either internal or external. A questionnaire was developed using these components of the model and administered to 191 diploma nursing students. An open-ended question asked students to list factors contributing to their success or failure in the nursing course they had just completed. Findings indicated that students generally used internal attributions to explain their successes and external attributions to explain their failures. Data obtained from the open-ended section of the questionnaire, however, showed that students rated faculty as the most significant reason for both success and failure. The faculty's availability and positive personality characteristics were most commonly correlated with the student's success, while the faculty's lack of skill or knowledge were most commonly associated with the student's failure.

Beginning nursing students typically feel overwhelmed and concerned about their ability to be successful in nursing. These feelings of anxiety and concern can have an adverse affect on students' academic performances and eventually their success in the nursing program. In an effort to determine the concerns of beginning nursing students, Williams (1993) surveyed 245 nursing students during their first week of study in a nursing program. An instrument was developed by the researcher and, after pilot testing, administered to the students. Content validity was established and reliability, as measured by Cronbach's alpha, was .93. Factor analysis yielded several areas of student concern. One area of concern was "faculty support and guidance." This factor contained items relating to students' concerns about "nonsupportive professors," "impatient professors," "not enough clinical guidance from professors," and "unclear expectations from professors." These items were ranked among the top 16 concerns identified by students. The top three items of concern identified by students were "keeping grades up," "fear of harming patient," and "learning clinical skills."

Certain student demographic characteristics were associated with higher levels of concern (Williams, 1993). Pearson correlations with selected demographic characteristics showed that being Asian was positively correlated ($p < .001$) with higher levels of concern related to support and guidance. Of the 245 nursing students who participated in this study, 23% identified themselves as Asian. Single marital status also was positively ($p < .001$) correlated with higher levels of concern related to support and guidance. It should be noted that the Pearson correlation coefficient is appropriate for use whenever the variables being measured are of an interval or ratio nature. Nonparametric tests are usually applied whenever the variables being measured are nominal in nature, as with gender, race, or ethnicity (Polit & Hungler, 1987). Multiple regression analyses also revealed that ethnicity was the most significant predictor of student concerns. Having an Asian ethnic background was a predictor for concern in the factor of support and guidance ($p < .0001$).

Williams' (1993) study addressed two major areas. First, it identified that the concerns of beginning nursing students, even at the very beginning of their educational experiences, are very similar to more experienced nursing students. Students begin their nursing programs with preconceived concerns about their relationships with faculty, coupled with serious concerns about developing their own level of competence. These preconceived concerns, if not acknowledged and addressed by faculty, can lead to dissatisfaction with the nursing program, increased levels of stress, and ultimately, withdrawal of the student from the program. Secondly, Williams' study identified ethnicity as an important variable that affects the concerns of beginning nursing students. It was recommended that faculty develop intervention strategies that will improve the cultural competence of faculty and provide students with orientation and support groups.

Sherrod et al. (1992) conducted interviews with 20 baccalaureate students to determine student perceptions of their academic and nonacademic experiences after completion of their first year in nursing school. Positive academic experiences included faculty guidance and support, and academic support services. Cited academic problems included excessive amount of content to learn, large classes, and faculty-related problems. The investigators suggested that attention should be given to student perceptions of their experiences in order to develop effective retention programs. The findings of this study tend to indicate that the role of the faculty advisor is a pivotal one that should encompass more than the traditional course scheduling advice (Sherrod et al., 1992).

RN-Students' Expectations of Student-Faculty Interactions

Registered nurses who return to school to pursue baccalaureate degrees may have different expectations of their interactions with faculty then do generic undergraduate students. Research has indicated that RN students desire learning environments that promote student autonomy, independence, acknowledgment of previously acquired competencies, and supportive faculty interactions.

Using an open-ended questionnaire, Baker and Barlow (1988) surveyed 89 RN students enrolled in a self-paced baccalaureate program in an attempt to evaluate a flexible option completion program and to identify characteristics that were associated with student success. Content analysis of the responses was used to identify the common factors of success listed by the students. The students identified motivation and determination, family support, and economic support as essential personal factors contributing to their academic success. They also identified essential faculty characteristics that contributed to their success, including encouraging student progress; being supportive and available to students; acknowledging the student's background; being considerate, caring, and friendly; and treating the students as peers and individuals. It is interesting to note that these RN students mentioned the importance of collegial, supportive faculty interactions contributing to their success four times as often as they mentioned the importance of faculty being knowledgeable. Limitations of this study included the use of a nonrandomized, convenience sample and lack of information regarding the reliability of the content analysis.

Beeman (1988) surveyed 284 undergraduate and RN students in 12 undergraduate programs to compare the RN students' perceptions of how successful these programs were at meeting their learning needs. There was a total of 188 RN students included in this study, with 59 RN students enrolled in basic BSN programs and 129 RN students enrolled in RN-only BSN programs. The non-RN students ($n = 96$) were included as controls for the study. The Beeman Educational Environment Measure for Adult Nurses (BEEMAN) questionnaire was administered to all participants and the students were additionally asked to complete four open-ended questions. Reliabilities for the six scales on the BEEMAN questionnaire ranged from .92 to .65. Quantitative and qualitative analysis of the data indicated that students in the RN-only programs felt that they had high levels of independence in their programs while the RN students enrolled in basic BSN programs felt constrained. All students indicated that it was important to experience environmental support from faculty and peers. Beeman concluded that it is faculty's willingness to support individualized learning needs, especially for RN students enrolled in basic BSN programs, that can determine the difference between success or failure for RN students.

It has been acknowledged that returning RNs frequently have different learning needs from generic BSN student. It is also important to determine if RN students have different stressors affecting them when they return to school. Lee (1987) attempted to identify and rank stressful clinical and didactic incidents experienced by returning RN students. Senior RN students ($n = 111$) from 10 schools of nursing were asked to describe a stressful incident that they had experienced during the past school year. The content of the responses was coded and analyzed. Reliability of the category codes was established using 3 independent coders. Students identified 67 stressful didactic incidents and 40 stressful clinical incidents. Inadequate instruction and instructor relations were subcategories of stress in both clinical and didactic categories with the mean amounts of stress in these subcategories ranging from 5.3 to 5.8 on a scale of 7.0. Since definitions of the various categories and the frequency with which the incidents occurred were not provided, it is not possible to further analyze the significance of these results.

Student-Faculty Interactions in Graduate Education

Supporting articles in the literature indicate that student-faculty interactions are an important contributing factor to the achievement of successful outcomes in graduate education. Meleis, Hall, and Stevens (1994), however, stated that the notion of caring in student-faculty relationships, as emphasized at the undergraduate level of education, is not sufficient for doctoral education. Instead, they offered the concept of "scholarly" caring that encompasses the importance of quality scholarship and knowledge base development, in addition to relational experiences. Collaborative mentorship, in which faculty and students directly work together on academic projects, is encouraged as a means of promoting student empowerment. The features of a collaborative mentorship would include negotiated relations, mutual interactions, and facilitative strategies for the professional development of each participant. This model of scholarly caring fosters the intellectual, sociocultural, and political competencies necessary at the graduate level.

Davidhizar (1988) also discussed mentoring in doctoral education. She stated that a mentoring relationship contributes to the development of competent nursing professionals, and, without such a relationship, doctoral education is incomplete. Davidhizar proposed that certain characteristics should exist in the mentoring relationship. These characteristics include an orientation toward the future, the presence of a common interest, development of strategies and advice for goal attainment, self-disclosure, and affirmation. However, Davidhizar did not explicitly address the idea of faculty being mentors for doctoral students.

While the literature seems to support the concept that interpersonal interactions with faculty can have an impact on graduate students' professional development and educational outcomes, research literature does not exist to support this assumption. It is also not possible to draw conclusions from the literature about the frequency with which graduate students are exposed to the concept of "scholarly caring" as defined by Meleis, Hall, and Stevens (1994).

Faculty Perceptions of Student-Faculty Interactions

While many studies have reported on student perceptions of student-faculty interactions, little research is available to describe how faculty view their interactions with students. Studies have been conducted, however, that allude to faculty perceptions of the importance of interpersonal relationships with students through comparisons with student perceptions. Students have consistently placed more importance on student-faculty interactions than do faculty. Most of these studies focused on the clinical faculty role.

In a descriptive, quantitative study, Stuebbe (1980) compared faculty and student perceptions of the role of the clinical instructor. The results indicated that students and faculty have different expectations of the clinical instructor's role. Students indicated that the nurse and person aspect of the role were most important, while faculty rated the teacher aspect of the role as most important. Reliability and validity of the tool used in this study were not reported. Brown conducted a similar study, comparing student ($n = 82$) and faculty ($n = 42$) descriptions of effective clinical teacher characteristics. Students perceived the teacher's interpersonal relationships with students to be more important than the teacher's professional competence, while faculty placed more importance on professional competence. Limitations of this study included the small sample size from only one institution and reliability of the tool was not reported.

Mogan and Knox (1987) surveyed 173 students and 28 clinical faculty to compare student and faculty perceptions of the characteristics of "best" and "worst" clinical faculty. Subjects were asked to recall their best and worst clinical instructors and rate them in the following areas: teaching ability, nursing competence, personality traits, interpersonal relationships, and evaluation. Students rated the interpersonal category higher than faculty ($p < .001$) when identifying "best" clinical teacher characteristics. There were no significant differences in perceptions of "worst" clinical teacher characteristics.

Pugh (1988) conducted a descriptive study to determine which clinical teaching behaviors faculty and students believed were most important. A questionnaire developed by the researcher was administered to 50 faculty and 358 students in eight BSN programs. Reliability of the tool was established for the faculty version of the questionnaire, but not the parallel student form. Findings indicated that faculty felt it was most important to provide students with positive reinforcement, encouragement with self-evaluation, and praise. Students, however, expressed the desire to have more empathetic, caring interactions with faculty than they were experiencing. Faculty admitted that they felt they operated in a closed-system, resulting in a sense of isolation within their clinical agencies. Faculty had few peers present to offer evaluation, guidance, or suggestions regarding their clinical teaching methodologies. Pugh stated that it may be difficult for faculty to develop positive interpersonal relationships with students if they themselves are not experiencing such relationships with their peers. It should be noted that 72% of the faculty surveyed in this study were still relatively new to teaching, with less than seven years of teaching experience. This raises the issue of how new faculty are socialized into their teaching roles.

Bergman and Gaitskill (1990), in their descriptive study of faculty and student perceptions of effective clinical teachers, reported an exception to the usual findings of students placing greater emphasis than faculty on interpersonal relations. In this study, both faculty ($n = 23$) and students ($n = 134$) valued skills related to faculty-student relationships over the professional or personal skills of the instructor. Findings suggested that displaying confidence and respect for the student were particularly important aspects of the student-faculty relationship. The authors suggested that clinical faculty should carefully consider the ethical dimensions of their interactions with students. Limitations to this study included the small sample size representing one institution.

Stephenson (1984) conducted an exploratory study in Britain using a grounded theory approach, as delineated by Glaser and Strauss (1967), to explore the expectations that students ($n = 22$) and faculty ($n = 23$) have of the student-faculty relationship. Findings indicated that both groups believed that faculty interacted with students in a caring fashion. However, there was a difference in agreement about the amount of social distance that should exist in the student-faculty relationship.

While faculty felt that a "certain amount" of social distance should exist between the two groups, only 50% of the students agreed. Faculty and students also disagreed on the type of relationship they experienced with each other; faculty felt the relationship with students was an informal one, while students felt the relationship was formal.

Other research has indicated that faculty and students perceive interactions differently. In a cross-sectional survey study conducted by Halstead (1993), a convenience sample of 104 baccalaureate senior nursing students and 45 baccalaureate nursing faculty from two schools of nursing completed a questionnaire measuring the perceived actual levels and desired levels of collegial communication present in their interactions with each other. Reliability and validity of the tool were established. Faculty reported higher perceived actual levels of collegiality than students ($p \leq .001$). There was a significant inverse relationship between student age and actual levels of collegiality experienced ($p < .05$). There was a significant positive relationship between age, years of experience as an RN, and the perceived actual levels of collegiality reported by faculty. Both groups desired higher levels of collegiality than were present in their interactions ($p \leq .001$). While faculty perceived they encouraged and demonstrated collegial behaviors with students, students did not necessarily perceive faculty to be highly collegial in their interactions. One implication of this study is that faculty may need to be more aware of how their interactions with students are being perceived by the students. Limitations of this study included the small sample size and reliance on self-reporting of behaviors.

DISCUSSION

The importance of student-faculty interactions cannot be underestimated by nurse educators. Careful thought should be given to designing learning experiences and promoting collegial learning environments that will foster the development of positive student-faculty relationships.

Despite the cited limitations of the research reviewed, students have consistently identified student-faculty interactions as having a significant impact on the quality of their educational experiences and their professional development. Research has primarily focused on student perceptions of student-faculty interactions at the undergraduate level. In studies that have compared student and faculty perceptions of student-faculty interactions, students have, with few exceptions, placed more emphasis on the significance of student-faculty interactions than have faculty. Faculty and students have also interpreted interactions differently.

It is evident that a lack of supportive, collegial relations with faculty can affect learning outcomes. No matter how knowledgeable faculty may be, if they do not relate positively to students, students may not hear the substance of the information being conveyed. This is an important concept to address in the development of the teaching role of faculty. Novice faculty, especially, need guidance in how to develop an effective interpersonal style with students.

The National League for Nursing (1993) has stated that there is a need to develop faculty-student relationships that are collaborative and egalitarian in nature. Before this can occur, however, the power relationships that exist in student-faculty relationships must be reconceptualized (Symonds, 1990). The teaching-learning process can be viewed as a process that results from the combined energies of both the student and the teacher. Empowerment results through the teaching process when the student-teacher exchanges are characterized by interaction, caring, commitment, creativity, and an acknowledgement of respect for the humanness of both student and teacher (Chally, 1992).

What kind of teaching strategies will most successfully move nursing education toward this concept of equity and empowerment in student-faculty relationships? Nursing education research has not yet addressed this issue. However, it is possible that learning experiences could be designed to encourage collaborative, collegial exchanges between faculty and students, between students, and between students, faculty, and nurses in practice settings. Examination of curricular content would reveal areas where discussion and examples of collegiality could be included and fostered through student-faculty interactions. Faculty participation in mentoring programs, academic advising, orientation programs, and student organizational activities are examples of how positive student-faculty interactions can be promoted outside the classroom or clinical settings.

Faculty should examine their own beliefs about the teaching-learning process and student-faculty interactions. Such an activity would help faculty gain an awareness of their own behaviors and attitudes. The classroom environment can be restructured so that the student becomes actively involved in the learning process, with less emphasis on the role of the educator as the sole determiner of learning experiences (Sellers & Haag, 1992). Clinical experiences can be designed to develop the self-confidence of students and enhance their participation as equal members of the health care team.

RECOMMENDATIONS FOR FUTURE RESEARCH

Research in the area of student-faculty interactions has primarily been exploratory and descriptive in nature. The sole reliance on quantitative methodology to examine student-faculty interactions has diminished. The number of qualitative, phenomenological studies about the lived experiences of nursing students has increased in recent years. The research has been consistent in establishing the importance of student-faculty interactions from the undergraduate student perspective. Research on graduate student perspectives and faculty perspectives of student-faculty interactions has been limited.

Research on the development of effective student-faculty interactions is minimal. The theoretical basis for the research conducted has frequently not been identified. Limitations in the research on student-faculty interactions most commonly included the use of small sample sizes, reliance on self-reporting of behaviors, and use of instruments without establishing reliability or validity.

In order to guide the future development of research in the area of student-faculty interactions, the following questions have been developed.

Students

- Do undergraduate students have different expectations of student-faculty interactions as they progress through their educational programs?
- What variables affect student perceptions of their interactions with faculty?
- How are perceptions of student-faculty interactions influenced by ethnicity?
- What expectations do graduate students have of student-faculty interactions?
- Are new graduates who have experienced supportive faculty-student interactions in their educational programs more successful in establishing collegial peer relationships in practice?

Faculty

- How do faculty develop their personal style of interactions with students?
- What factors affect faculty's ability to develop the level of positive student relationships that they desire?
- Are faculty who experience positive peer relationships more likely to establish such relationships with students?
- How do the power-sharing beliefs of faculty compare with their power-sharing actions?
- What strategies are most likely to be successful in increasing the cultural competence of faculty in their interactions with ethnically diverse student populations?

Teaching Methodologies

- What learning experiences are most successful in exposing students to the professional value of collegiality?
- What teaching strategies are most conducive to fostering positive student-faculty interactions?
- Does the quality of student-faculty interactions affect students' ability to develop critical thinking skills?
- How can students be helped to cope with the stress of being evaluated in the clinical setting?

Addressing these questions about student-faculty interactions, as well as others, through the development of theoretically grounded research will allow nurse educators to continue the reconceptualization of nursing curricula as a collaborative partnership between students and faculty.

REFERENCES

American Association of Colleges of Nursing. (1986). *Essentials of college and university education for professional nursing.* Washington, DC: Author.

Appleton, C. (1990). The meaning of human care and the experience of caring in a university school of nursing. In M. Leininger & J. Watson (Eds.), *The caring imperative in education* (pp. 77–93). New York: National League for Nursing Press.

Baker, S. S., & Barlow, D. J. (1988). Successful registered nurse education: A case analysis. *Nurse Educator, 13*(1), 18–22.

Beck, C. T. (1991). How students perceive faculty caring: A phenomenological study. *Nurse Educator, 16*(5), 18–22.

Beck, D. L., & Srivastava, R. (1991). Perceived level and sources of stress in baccalaureate nursing students. *Journal of Nursing Education, 30*(3), 127–133.

Beeman, P. (1988). RN's perceptions of their baccalaureate programs: Meeting their adult learning needs. *Journal of Nursing Education, 27*(8), 364–370.

Bergman, K., & Gaitskill, T. (1990). Faculty and student perceptions of effective clinical teachers: An extension study. *Journal of Professional Nursing, 6*(1), 33–44.

Betz, C. L. (1985). Students in transition: Imitators of role models. *Journal of Nursing Education, 24*(7), 301–303.

Brown, G. D. (1993). Accounting for power: Nurse teachers' and students' perceptions of power in their relationship. *Nurse Education Today, 13,* 111–120.

Brown, S. T. (1981). Faculty and student perceptions of effective clinical teachers. *Journal of Nursing Education, 20*(9), 4–15.

Chally, P. S. (1992). Empowerment through teaching. *Journal of Nursing Education, 31*(3), 117–120.

Davidhizar, R. E. (1988). Mentoring in doctoral education. *Journal of Advanced Nursing, 13*, 775–781.

Davidhizar, R. E., & McBride, A. (1985). How nursing students explain their success and failure in clinical experiences. *Journal of Nursing Education, 24*(7), 284–290.

Dixon, J. K., & Koerner, B. (1976). Faculty and student perceptions of effective classroom teaching in nursing. *Nursing Research, 25*(4), 300–305.

Flagler, S., Loper-Powers, S., & Spitzer, A. (1988). Clinical teaching is more than evaluation alone! *Journal of Nursing Education, 27*(8), 342–348.

Frank, B. (1994). Caring: Curricular issues. In L. R. Allen (Ed.), *Review of Research in Nursing Education, Volume VI* (pp. 33–56). New York: National League for Nursing Press.

Garrett, A., Manuel, D., & Vincent, C. (1976). Stressful experiences identified by student nurses. *Journal of Nursing Education, 15*(6), 9–18.

Glaser, B., & Strauss, A. (1967). *The discovery of a grounded theory.* London: Weidenfield & Nicholson.

Griffith, J. W., & Bakanauskas, A. J. (1983). Student-instructor relationships in nursing education. *Journal of Nursing Education, 22*(3), 104–107.

Halldorsdottir, S. (1990). The essential structure of a caring and an uncaring encounter with a teacher: The perspective of the nursing student. In M. Leininger & J. Watson (Eds.), *The caring imperative in education* (pp. 95–107). New York: National League for Nursing Press.

Halstead, J. A. (1993). The extent of collegiality in student-faculty interactions as perceived by baccalaureate nursing students and faculty. *Proceedings and Abstracts of the 1993 11th Annual Conference on Research in Nursing Education, Council for the Society for Research in Nursing Education, National League for Nursing Press*, p. 30.

Hammer, R. M., & Tufts, M. A. (1985). Nursing student's self image—nursing educator's responsibilities. *Journal of Nursing Education, 24*(7), 280–283.

Hughes, L. (1992). Faculty-student interactions and the student-perceived climate for caring. *Advances in Nursing Science, 14*(3), 60–71.

Jacox, A. (1978). Professional socialization of nurses. In N. Chaska (Ed.), *The nursing profession: Views through the mist* (pp. 10–19). New York: McGraw-Hill.

Jones, S. L., & Jones, P. K. (1977). Nursing student definitions of the "real" nurse. *Journal of Nursing Education, 16*(4), 15–21.

Kelly, B. (1992). The professional self-concepts of nursing undergraduates and their perceptions of influential forces. *Journal of Nursing Education, 31*(3), 121–125.

Kleehammer, K., Hart, A. L., & Keck, J. F. (1990). Nursing students' perceptions of anxiety-producing situations in the clinical setting. *Journal of Nursing Education, 29*(4), 183–187.

Kramer, M. (1968). Role models, role conceptions, and role deprivation. *Nursing Research, 17*(2), 115–120.

Kushnir, T. (1986). Stress and social facilitation: The effects of the presence of an instructor on student nurses' behaviour. *Journal of Advanced Nursing, 11,* 13–19.

Layton, M. M. (1969). How instructors' attitudes affect students. *Nursing Outlook, 17*(1), 27–29.

Lee, E. J. (1987). Analysis of stressful clinical and didactic incidents reported by returning registered nurses. *Journal of Nursing Education, 26*(9), 372–378.

Meleis, A. I., Hall, J. M., & Stevens, P. (1994). Scholarly caring in doctoral nursing education: Promoting diversity and collaborative mentorship. *Image: Journal of Nursing Scholarship, 26*(3), 177–180.

Miller, B. K., Haber, J., & Byrne, M. W. (1990). The experience of caring in the teaching-learning process of nursing education: Student and teacher perspectives. In M. Leininger & J. Watson (Eds.), *The caring imperative in education* (pp. 125–135). New York: National League of Nursing Press.

Mogan, J., & Knox, J. E. (1987). Characteristics of "best" and "worst" clinical teachers as perceived by university nursing faculty and students. *Journal of Advanced Nursing, 12,* 331–337.

National League for Nursing. (1993). *A vision for nursing education.* New York: Author.

Nelms, T. P. (1990). The lived experience of nursing education: A phenomenological study. In M. Leininger & J. Watson (Eds.), *The caring imperative in education* (pp. 285–297). New York: National League for Nursing Press.

O'Reilly-Knapp, M. (1994). Reports by baccalaureate nursing students of social support. *IMAGE: Journal of Nursing Scholarship, 26*(2), 139–142.

Pagana, K. D. (1988). Stresses and threats reported by baccalaureate students in relation to an initial clinical experience. *Journal of Nursing Education, 27*(9), 418–424.

Polit, D., & Hungler, B. (1987). *Nursing research: Principles and methods.* Philadelphia: Lippincott.

90 Judith A. Halstead

Pugh, E. J. (1988). Soliciting student input to improve clinical teaching. *Nurse Educator, 13*(5), 28–33.

Rather, M. L. (1994). Schooling for oppression: A critical hermeneutical analysis of the lived experience of the returning RN student. *Journal of Nursing Education, 33*(6), 263–271.

Schaffer, M. A., & Juarez, M. (1993). An ethical analysis of student-faculty interactions. *Nurse Educator, 18*(3), 25–28.

Sellers, S. C., & Haag, B. A. (1992). Achieving equity in nursing education. *Nursing & Health Care, 13*(3), 134–137.

Sherrod, R. A., Harrison, L. L., Lowery, B. H., Wood, F. G., Edwards, R. M., Gaskins, S. W., & Buttram, T. (1992). Freshmen baccalaureate nursing students' perceptions of their academic and nonacademic experiences: Implications for retention. *Journal of Professional Nursing, 8*(4), 203–208.

Stephenson, P. M. (1984). Aspects of the nurse tutor-student nurse relationship. *Journal of Advanced Nursing, 9,* 283–290.

Stuebbe, B. (1980). Student and faculty perspectives on the role of a nursing instructor. *Journal of Nursing Education, 19*(7), 4–9.

Symonds, J. M. (1990). Revolutionizing the student-teacher relationship. In *Curriculum revolution: Redefining the student-teacher relationship* (pp. 47–55). New York: National League for Nursing Press.

Theis, E. C. (1988). Nursing students' perspectives of unethical teaching behaviors. *Journal of Nursing Education, 27*(3), 102–106.

Williams, R. (1993). The concerns of beginning nursing students. *Nursing and Health Care, 14*(4), 178–184.

Wilson, M. (1994). Nursing student perspectives of learning in a clinical setting. *Journal of Nursing Education, 33*(2), 81–86.

Windsor, A. (1987). Nursing students' perceptions of clinical experience. *Journal of Nursing Education, 26*(4), 150–154.

Wong, S. (1978). Nurse-teacher behaviours in the clinical field: Apparent effect on nursing students' learning. *Journal of Advanced Nursing, 3,* 369–372.

Chapter Four

RESEARCH ON TEACHING IN THE CLINICAL SETTING
Marilyn H. Oermann, PhD, RN, FAAN

Clinical practice in nursing education programs provides the means for students to develop knowledge, cognitive and technological skills, and a value system for care of clients. Through their clinical experiences, students learn effective methods of reasoning and approaching patient problems and become socialized into the profession. Such outcomes may be achieved in any setting in which students are involved in the practice of nursing. While clinical practice in nursing programs occurred traditionally in hospitals and public health settings, a shift toward the community—to prepare students for practice in community-based systems (de Tornyay, 1993; Oermann, 1994a, 1994b; Reilly & Oermann, 1992)—is gaining ground. Regardless of the setting for clinical practice, though, the teacher plays a decisive role in developing meaningful experiences for students, so as to achieve prescribed outcomes and prepare students for present and future practice.

This review includes research on clinical teaching from 1965 to 1995. The *Cumulative Nursing Index* was searched manually and an automated bibliographic search was conducted to obtain studies for analysis. The table of contents of relevant nursing journals, such as the *Journal of Nursing Education,* also were examined. To be included in the review, the research needed to: (1) focus on clinical teaching within a nursing education program; (2) represent empirical studies not descriptions of a particular clinical experience; (3) report the research design, sample, methodology, and results; and (4) represent studies with students in diploma, associate degree (ADN), baccalaureate (BSN), or graduate nursing programs. One-hundred thirty-four studies were identified, and based on these criteria, 94 were reviewed.

The research was divided into four major classifications; the number of studies reviewed in each category is indicated: (1) teacher behaviors in the clinical setting ($n = 27$); (2) clinical teaching methods including patient assignment, written assignments, clinical conference, observation, media used in the clinical setting, and preceptorships ($n = 46$);

(3) student perceptions of clinical (n = 10); and (4) the clinical experience in general (n = 11). Among the research reviewed, study designs were predominantly descriptive, involving surveys of students, and quasi-experimental. A few of the more recent studies used qualitative methods. In general, investigators surveyed students in one setting only. Sample sizes ranged from 7 to 487; in many studies, a major limitation was the small sample size. Outcome variables included predominantly clinical performance, cognitive learning, self-confidence, student satisfaction, role development, and stress; other outcome variables were unique to the particular research. Questionnaires, rating scales, written tests, case studies, tape recordings, and observational techniques were used for data collection.

TEACHER BEHAVIORS IN CLINICAL SETTING

The majority of research on clinical teaching focused on characteristics and qualities of the teacher. While a larger number of studies on teaching methods (n = 46) were found, this category included a wide range of instructional methods grouped together for the purposes of the review; none of the methods was studied individually to the same extent as was teaching effectiveness. Twenty-seven studies addressed teacher behaviors in the clinical setting. This research began in the 1960s and has continued through the present. The review presented in this section of the chapter builds on an earlier one by Pugh (1983) in the first volume of *Review of Research in Nursing Education*. Most of the studies have been completed since Pugh's (1983) review, reflecting continued interest in this topic.

In part of the chapter, individual studies are critiqued and their findings are synthesized as they relate to overall qualities of effective clinical teaching in nursing. Broad generalizations about teaching effectiveness in nursing are made from the research findings. In the remaining sections of the chapter, limitations of the research and an insufficient number of studies make it difficult to derive a similar set of generalizations; for this reason, each study is described individually.

Knowledge and Clinical Competence

Across studies, students describe an effective clinical teacher as knowledgeable and willing to share that knowledge and expertise with them in the clinical setting (Armington, Reinikka, & Creighton, 1972; Bergman & Gaitskill, 1990; Brown, 1981; Mogan & Knox, 1987; Nehring, 1990; Windsor, 1987). This knowledge includes an understanding of theories and concepts used in practice and ability to assist students in applying them to clinical practice (Bergman & Gaitskill, 1990; Brown, 1981; Pugh, 1988).

Using a descriptive design, Brown (1981) compared perceptions of clinical teaching effectiveness between senior nursing students ($n = 82$) and faculty ($n = 42$) from one baccalaureate program. Brown's questionnaire identified 20 characteristics of clinical teachers to which respondents rated their importance on a Likert scale. While differences existed between students and faculty in their descriptions of effective clinical teachers, both groups emphasized the importance of the teacher being well-informed, able to communicate that knowledge to students, and objective and fair in evaluation. A related behavior was the ability to assist students in applying theory to practice. Respecting students, conveying confidence in them, and encouraging them to ask questions were other important clinical teacher behaviors.

Bergman and Gaitskill (1990), using a descriptive design, extended this earlier study by Brown (1981). Brown's questionnaire was distributed to 134 baccalaureate nursing students and 23 faculty in a midwest university. Data were analyzed with the same method used by Brown, providing for generalizations across studies. Both students and faculty identified the need for the teacher to be articulate and knowledgeable. Objectivity and fairness in evaluation and ability to provide useful feedback were other important teacher behaviors. The importance of a positive student-faculty relationship in the clinical setting was recognized by both groups of subjects. The 20 characteristics of clinical teacher effectiveness were categorized in terms of relationships with students, professional competence, and personal attributes of the teacher. In the earlier study by Brown (1981), however, faculty ranked professional competence above relationships with students.

The teacher's theoretical and clinical knowledge used in practice has been labeled nursing competence by some researchers (Knox & Mogan, 1985; Mogan & Knox, 1987; Nehring, 1990). Findings of their research indicate that this nursing competence is an important characteristic of clinical teaching effectiveness. In the early study, Knox and Mogan (1985) developed a 47-item instrument describing clinical teacher characteristics; reliability coefficients ranged from .70 to .89. The instrument was distributed to 666 subjects including students and faculty in a university school of nursing in Western Canada and graduates of the program. Of those distributed, 487 (73%) were returned. All three groups of respondents ranked evaluation as most important among the characteristics of teaching effectiveness. Similar perceptions of teacher effectiveness were found across the groups.

In 1987, Mogan and Knox compared characteristics of the best and worst clinical teachers as perceived by students and faculty. Building on their earlier research, the investigators distributed the Nursing Clinical

Teacher Effectiveness Inventory (NCTEI), a 48-item checklist on individual teacher characteristics, to 173 BSN students and 28 clinical faculty. The alpha coefficient was .79 to .92; test-retest reliability ranged from .76 to .93. The NCTEI is one of the instruments in this area with reported validity and reliability. Both students and faculty agreed that being a good role model was the most important characteristic of effective clinical teaching.

Nehring (1990) conducted a follow-up of Mogan and Knox's (1987) study exploring the best and worst clinical teachers as perceived by both faculty and students. In Nehring's research, 63 baccalaureate nursing faculty and 121 students completed the NCTEI. Subjects described the best clinical teacher as being a good role model, enjoying teaching and nursing, and demonstrating clinical skills and judgment. Serving as a role model and encouraging mutual respect between teacher and student were two characteristics which distinguished the best and worst clinical faculty.

Clinical Competence of Teacher

Effective clinical teaching also requires competence in clinical practice. Nehring (1990) found, similar to the earlier study by Mogan and Knox (1987), that the best teachers demonstrated expert clinical skills and judgment. The importance of maintaining clinical competence has been reported in other studies (Bergman & Gaitskill, 1990; Brown, 1981; Kiker, 1973; Pugh, 1988; Rauen, 1974; Sieh & Bell, 1994).

Rauen (1974) in an early study of role characteristics of clinical nurse teachers found that the teacher's skill in demonstrating how to function in a real nursing situation was important. In Rauen's study, freshman and senior nursing students ($n = 84$) in three diploma programs were questioned as to whether they expected the clinical faculty to serve as a role model. Rauen identified the clinical instructor as serving three roles: teacher, nurse, and person. Using this as a framework, she developed the Clinical Instructor Characteristics Ranking Scale (CICRS) for use in the research. The CICRS consists of 18 characteristics of the clinical teacher with an equal number of teacher, nurse, and person behaviors. Students indicated that nurse role characteristics were more important than teacher and person roles.

In a replication of Rauen's study, Stuebbe (1980) examined how students view the role of the clinical instructor and compared this with the teacher's own view of this role. Sixty-eight students and 12 faculty from a diploma program completed the CICRS. Faculty ranked teacher characteristics highest and students ranked nurse characteristics highest.

Pugh (1988) compared clinical teaching behaviors identified as important by both teachers ($n = 50$) and students ($n = 358$) in eight randomly selected BSN programs. Using a questionnaire with 20 teacher behaviors, faculty and students rated the importance of these behaviors for student learning. The most important characteristics identified by faculty were showing genuine interest in students, giving feedback on written assignments, encouraging self-evaluation, and giving positive reinforcement and praise in the clinical setting. Students reported that effective teachers are ones who demonstrate nursing care in a real situation, give feedback on written assignments and for own improvement in clinical, and facilitate students' meeting own learning goals. While students rated the teacher's ability to demonstrate nursing care in a real situation as most important, this was not ranked as high by faculty respondents.

The ability to demonstrate care in a real situation was confirmed in research by Horst (1988). Junior and senior nursing students ($n = 183$) completed the CICRS developed originally by Rauen (1974). The three highest ranking characteristics among these subjects were ability to demonstrate care in a real nursing situation, enthusiasm for providing quality patient care, and availability in the clinical setting for student assistance.

There is sufficient research to conclude that two important dimensions of clinical teaching effectiveness are the teacher's knowledge about the practice area in which teaching and own clinical competence. While the research is inconsistent on the ranking of these characteristics in comparison with other important teaching behaviors, it is clear that effective clinical teaching requires a knowledgeable and competent faculty who is able to communicate that knowledge to students.

Teaching Practices and Skill

Skill in teaching involves the ability of the teacher to diagnose learning needs, plan instruction which reflects student needs and the goals of the clinical experience, supervise students effectively, and evaluate learning. Ability to plan assignments that help in transfer of learning to the clinical setting was rated as an important characteristic of teaching effectiveness by faculty in Pugh's study (1988). Findings from research suggest that the best clinical teachers are good role models for students, enjoy teaching, are well-prepared for teaching, stimulate student interest, explain concepts and procedures clearly, demonstrate effective clinical skills and judgment, and supervise students effectively (Armington, Reinikka, & Creighton, 1972; Barham, 1965; Bergman & Gaitskill, 1990; Mims, 1970; Mogan & Knox, 1987; Nehring, 1990; Pugh, 1988; Reeve, 1994; Windsor, 1987; Wiseman, 1994).

In an early study, Barham (1965) used a critical incident technique to identify important clinical teaching behaviors. Effective teachers give clear explanations, are available to students in clinical, and stimulate them to learn. In Windsor's study (1987), students identified the need for clinical faculty to have high expectations of them in clinical, assign difficult tasks, and encourage them to solve problems.

The purpose of a study by Wiseman (1994) was to describe role modeling behaviors of the clinical faculty. Using Bandura's Social Learning Theory as a framework, she developed a questionnaire on 28 role model behaviors. The alpha coefficient was .95. Data were collected from 208 BSN students in three schools of nursing. Juniors and seniors ranked the role model behaviors of faculty similarly. Wiseman (1994) concluded that students consider clinical faculty as role models.

Krichbaum (1994) explored the relationship between 24 clinical teacher behaviors used by critical care preceptors ($n = 36$) in their teaching and achievement of learning outcomes by their BSN students ($n = 36$). Two measures of learning were used: performance in the clinical setting as measured by a clinical evaluation instrument and performance on a standardized test of critical care knowledge, the Basic Knowledge Assessment Tool (BKAT). Each preceptor's use of clinical teaching behaviors was assessed by the preceptors themselves and students using similar instruments. Coefficient alphas on these instruments ranged from .92 to .93. Correlations were computed between clinical teacher effectiveness ratings and student learning as measured by increased scores on the BKAT. Student learning was significantly related to specific teaching skills of the preceptor, including use of objectives for clinical teaching, providing opportunities for practice, asking appropriate questions, and providing specific and timely feedback. There were significant correlations between student performance in clinical and the preceptor's ability to modify expectations based on the learner's level of performance, clarity in the way in which the clinical practicum was structured, opportunities provided for observing nurses in practice, appropriateness of the preceptor's questions, and extent of feedback given to students. This is one of the few studies in which specific learning outcomes are linked to teaching practices; further research is needed to substantiate these findings.

Other studies emphasize the importance of the teacher's skill and practices in clinical evaluation. Findings confirm that positive and useful feedback on student progress is an important characteristic of effective clinical teaching (Bergman & Gaitskill, 1990; Krichbaum, 1994; Nehring, 1990; O'Shea & Parsons, 1979; Pugh, 1988; Windsor, 1987). Other evaluative practices of the clinical teacher which influence teaching effectiveness include using and sharing anecdotal notes with students (Pugh, 1988), exhibiting fairness in evaluation (Bergman & Gaitskill, 1990; Jacobson, 1966), promoting student independence through evaluative practices, correcting mistakes without belittling students, communicating clear expectations to learners (Nehring, 1990; O'Shea & Parsons, 1979; Sieh & Bell, 1994), and encouraging self-evaluation (Pugh, 1988).

O'Shea and Parsons (1979) collected data on clinical teacher effectiveness from 205 students and 24 faculty in a baccalaureate nursing program by asking subjects to list 3 to 5 teacher behaviors that facilitated their learning in the clinical setting and a similar number of behaviors which inhibited their learning. Responses of students were categorized as evaluative behaviors, assistive behaviors, and personal characteristics. The importance of providing positive and honest feedback was identified by both students and faculty as facilitating learning in the clinical setting. Insufficient and only negative feedback impeded learning. Instructional behaviors which facilitated learning in clinical included availability in the clinical setting and willingness to help students in practice. Supportive and understanding behaviors of the teacher also facilitated student learning.

The importance of the teacher providing positive, honest, and frequent feedback to students in clinical practice is evident in the research. Flagler, Loper-Powers, and Spitzer (1988) found that giving positive reinforcement and specific feedback as well as encouraging questions, showing confidence in the student, and supporting the student in clinical were instructor behaviors which enhanced students' development of self-confidence as a nurse. Similarly, giving no feedback or only negative feedback hindered their self-confidence in practice. In their study, 139 baccalaureate nursing students rated 16 clinical teaching behaviors as to whether they helped or hindered the student's development of self-confidence as a nurse. The questionnaire used for the rating, however, was not tested for validity and reliability, a limitation of the study. Factor analysis revealed five factors accounting for 96% of the variance. These factors reflect dimensions of the clinical teacher role: resource person, evaluator, encourager, promoter of patient care, and benevolent presence.

Sieh and Bell (1994), in research with 199 students and 22 faculty from two community colleges, found that the highest ranked characteristic of effective clinical teaching as perceived by students was correcting their mistakes without belittling them. Not criticizing students in front of others was ranked third. Characteristics ranked high by faculty included encouraging a climate of mutual respect, giving specific suggestions for improvement and constructive feedback, and correcting student mistakes without belittling them. The investigators used a descriptive design; data were collected with the NCTEI. This recent study on teaching effectiveness used a validated instrument rather than one developed by the investigators for their particular study; involved a large sample of ADN students; and included more than one setting, thereby improving generalizability.

The need for the teacher to be available to students in the clinical setting has been reported in some of the research. Reeve (1994) found that less experienced students believed it was more important for faculty to be available and to assist them than seniors, advanced placement RNs, and new graduates. Availability to work with students in clinical as the situation arises also was reported by Bergman and Gaitskill (1990). Students in the study by Flagler, Loper-Powers, and Spitzer (1988) indicated that availability of the instructor in clinical was an important behavior that promoted their development of self-confidence.

Findings from the research suggest that there are specific teaching skills needed by the faculty in the clinical setting. The best clinical teachers plan assignments which reflect student needs and promote transfer of learning to the clinical setting, are good role models, give clear explanations, effectively demonstrate procedures and clinical skills, exhibit fairness in evaluation, and give positive and consistent feedback, among other behaviors. Further research similar to Krichbaum's (1994) study is needed to establish the relationship between clinical teacher behaviors and measurable learning outcomes.

Interpersonal Relationships with Students

The ability of the clinical instructor to interact with students is another important teacher behavior. This skill, identified early on by Jacobson (1966) and confirmed throughout the research, involves interacting with students on a one-to-one basis and as a group. Bergman and Gaitskill (1990) found that among different characteristics of effective clinical teaching interpersonal relationships with students were ranked as most important. These characteristics included conveying confidence in and respect for students, having realistic expectations of them, being honest and direct, and encouraging students to ask questions and participate freely in discussions. In Nehring's (1990) research, the best clinical teachers as perceived by both faculty and students were approachable, encouraged mutual respect, and provided support and encouragement to learners. Other studies have confirmed the importance of interpersonal relations with students in clinical teaching (Brown, 1981; Krichbaum, 1994; Mogan & Knox, 1987; Pugh, 1988; Reeve, 1994).

Karns and Schwab (1982) examined nursing students' perceptions of teaching behaviors which promoted positive relationships in clinical between faculty and students. Findings suggested that empathy, genuiness, and respect for learners were important dimensions of this interpersonal relationship.

In Beck's (1991) phenomenological study of student perceptions of faculty caring, 47 incidents of a caring student-faculty experience were analyzed; only 8 of these occurred in the clinical setting. This caring experience between faculty and students reflected three clusters of themes: attentive presence, sharing of selves, and consequences of the experience in which the student feels respected and valued.

Teaching is an interactional process dependent on the teacher's ability to develop effective relationships with learners. While important for teaching in any setting, this interpersonal dimension is critical for teaching in the clinical setting (Reilly & Oermann, 1992). Findings from the research confirm the importance of developing a positive relationship with the student in clinical. Characteristics of effective teaching in this area include, among others, conveying respect for the student, being honest, and providing support and encouragement. While the notion of a caring relationship is implicit throughout the research, Beck (1991) describes in greater depth student perceptions of a caring student-faculty experience; this line of research should be continued.

Personal Characteristics of Teacher

One last dimension important in clinical teaching effectiveness relates to the personal attributes and characteristics of the teacher. In the study by O'Shea and Parsons (1979), friendly, supportive, and understanding behaviors of the clinical teacher promoted learning. In more recent studies, while described differently in the research, these characteristics include enthusiasm, a sense of humor, willingness to admit limitations and mistakes honestly, cooperation and patience, and flexibility in the clinical setting (Bergman & Gaitskill, 1990; Mogan & Knox, 1987; Nehring, 1990). Promoting freedom of discussion and providing an opportunity to vent feelings also were reported by Brown (1981) as important behaviors of the teacher.

Students in Pugh's study (1988) rated as important giving encouragement and praise to students and showing an interest in them. These same two behaviors were ranked even higher by faculty. Flagler, Loper-Powers, and Spitzer (1988) suggest that these teacher behaviors are beneficial to the student's development of self-confidence. In Krichbaum's study (1994), the enthusiasm of the preceptor and concern for the learner correlated significantly with students' performance in clinical practice and cognitive outcomes.

The majority of studies on clinical teaching suggest that the personal characteristics of the teacher may influence teaching effectiveness although differences exist in how they are described. One characteristic identified consistently in the research, though, is the teacher's enthusiasm. An enthusiastic faculty is important in students' evaluations of effective clinical teaching and may influence their performance and cognitive outcomes as suggested by Krichbaum (1994); further study of the effect of enthusiasm on specific learning outcomes is indicated. One limitation of the research on teaching effectiveness is the lack of control for the teacher's age, years of experience, and other characteristics of the individual faculty which may influence the results particularly with this personal dimension.

Instruments for Measuring Clinical Teacher Effectiveness

The intent of four other studies was to develop and test instruments for measuring clinical teaching effectiveness. These studies were categorized separately because their purpose was instrument development alone.

The purpose of Zimmerman and Westfall's (1988) study was to develop and validate the Effective Teaching Clinical Behaviors (ETCB) scale and establish its validity and reliability. A convenience sample of 281 students from three nursing programs, two BSN and one diploma, evaluated 29 clinical faculty using the ETCB. Factor analysis suggested that the instrument measured one factor, effective clinical teaching behavior. Cronbach's alpha was .97; test-retest reliability for both forms of the ETCB was .93 to .94. Findings established the validity and reliability of the instrument; replication with different levels of students and across settings is warranted.

Fong and McCauley (1993) assessed the content validity, construct validity, internal consistency, and test-retest reliability of the Clinical Teaching Evaluation (CTE) instrument. Content validity was established by 14 faculty teaching in a BSN program who confirmed the appropriateness of each item in the instrument. Factor analysis using a principle component method revealed three factors that accounted for 64% of the total variance: nursing competence, consideration for students, and teaching competence. Undergraduate students ($n = 384$) used the CTE for evaluation of 27 clinical instructors. Cronbach's alpha was .97 indicating high internal consistency; Pearson's correlation was high between the first administration of the instrument and retest ($r = .85$, $p < .001$). While further studies are indicated with different subjects and settings, this research was important in developing valid and reliable instruments for evaluating teaching effectiveness.

Reeve (1994) also described the development and testing of an instrument to measure clinical teacher effectiveness in a series of well-designed pilot studies. In the first phase of testing, 50 characteristics of effective teaching were identified by the investigator and reviewed by faculty from one BSN program. The characteristics were then grouped into categories of effective clinical teaching as identified in the literature. Faculty ($n = 42$), BSN students ($n = 420$), and recent program graduates ($n = 142$) rated on a five-point Likert scale the importance of each characteristic. Criteria were established to reduce the number of characteristics in the instrument to 27 items. The pilot test with students ($n = 205$) at the end of their clinical courses provided beginning validation of the instrument. While demographic data were collected from both students and teachers, the investigator does not report the influence, if any, of these demographic variables.

Much of the research on clinical teachers in nursing uses a quantitative methodology involving surveys of students and faculty. Mogan and Warbinek (1994), however, reported on the development and initial psychometric testing of an instrument to observe and record teaching behaviors of clinical faculty. The Observations of Nursing Teachers in Clinical Setting (ONTICS) consists of 44 items on effective and ineffective teacher behaviors grouped in nine categories. The researchers observed 12 volunteer clinical teachers across five hospitals in Canada for two consecutive hours recording their observations of the teacher. Following each observation, the researchers then categorized the teacher behaviors. The researchers concluded that this instrument for observing teacher behaviors appears to capture an aspect of clinical teaching effectiveness not measured through surveys and other more subjective instruments.

Developing valid and reliable measures of clinical teaching effectiveness remains an important goal. The instruments described in this section were developed from the literature and prior research; these initial studies document their validity and reliability. Further testing is warranted, however, with larger samples, varying levels of nursing students, different types of nursing programs, and multiple settings. Rather than continuing to develop new instruments, researchers should test and revise existing ones.

Role of Clinical Teacher

While some of the research on clinical teacher effectiveness also addresses the role of the faculty, three other studies focused on different dimensions of the teacher's role in the clinical setting irrespective of specific teacher behaviors and characteristics. The effect of faculty practice on the role of the teacher was examined by Kramer, Polifroni, and Organek (1986). The sample included 134 senior BSN students and 14 faculty teaching them in the clinical setting. Students taught by faculty in practice scored higher in three areas: integrating theory into practice, possessing a realistic perception of the work environment, and cooperating and participating in nursing research. In addition, these students had a higher degree of autonomy, higher self-concept and self-esteem, and more professional and bicultural role behaviors than students taught by faculty not in practice.

In a qualitative study, Morgan (1991) explored the teaching activities that clinical instructors used during actual clinical teaching and ones they would use in response to a scenario of a clinical teaching event. The investigator interviewed nine randomly selected clinical faculty in a BSN program. The usual teaching activities identified by these faculty were role modelling and demonstration. Replication of this study is needed with clinical teachers from varied programs and teaching different levels of students. Teaching activities for beginning students may be different from other levels of learners and may vary considerably across clinical practice areas.

Piscopo (1994) examined role strain among clinical nursing faculty. The sample included 31 faculty teaching in BSN programs in one geographic setting and the nursing manager from the unit in which they had students. Multiple instruments were used to measure organizational climate, communication within the organization, and role strain. There was no significant difference between perceptions of the faculty and nurse manager of organizational climate although there were significant differences between these groups in perception of communication in the organization. Nurse managers had a more positive perception of communication within the clinical agency (t[60] = 3.95, $p < .01$). Piscopo (1994) suggested that the difference in perceptions of communication may be related to the fact that faculty are not members of the organization and as such are not part of the formal communication network. Because faculty spend a designated amount of time in the setting, they may not understand fully the communication channels within the organization.

Further study is needed to more clearly describe the role and instructional activities of the teacher in clinical; stresses experienced by clinical faculty; and role of part-time, adjunct, and other types of faculty who teach nursing students. Other questions not answered in the research deal with the preparation of faculty for clinical teaching, supervision and mentoring of new instructors, providing support for faculty in the clinical setting, and impact of turnover of clinical faculty on the program and quality of teaching.

Summary

Considering the research on clinical teaching in nursing, studies on teacher effectiveness dominate. Results of these studies suggest behaviors of effective clinical teachers in nursing which are consistent with research in other health professions and higher education in general. While there are differences across studies, generalizations may be drawn from this research. Effective clinical teaching reflects the teacher's knowledge of nursing, clinical competence, teaching practices and skill in the instructional process, ability to develop interpersonal relationships with students individually and as a group, and personal characteristics such as enthusiasm, flexibility, and a sense of humor. Limitations of the research include small sample sizes in some of the studies; the use of convenience samples of students and faculty typically from one setting only and BSN programs; need for further testing of instruments; lack of assessment of teaching effectiveness across clinical courses, practice areas, and types of clinical settings; lack of control of individual teacher characteristics which might influence teaching effectiveness, such as, age, prior teaching and clinical experience, and specialty area; and characteristics of the student that might be significant, such as, age, gender, prior educational and work experience, and level in the program. The influence of these individual characteristics, if any, has not been studied. It also is important to note that the research focuses predominantly on BSN students; few studies were done with ADN students and none at the graduate level. More than a decade ago, Pugh (1983) identified many of the same limitations in terms of sampling and recommended that studies be replicated with different groups of students in multiple settings.

Although much of the research reflects one-time studies, a number of investigators have extended earlier research (Bergman & Gaitskill, 1990; Horst, 1988; Nehring, 1990; Pugh, 1988; Stuebbe, 1980). Steubbe (1980) and Horst (1988) replicated Rauen's (1974) early study, providing an opportunity to examine clinical teaching behaviors with different students and settings but measured by the same instrument. Other investigators have built upon earlier research which is important to develop a body of knowledge about clinical teaching. Bergman and Gaitskill (1990) replicated Brown's (1981) study in a different geographic area and with varying levels of nursing students. Brown's questionnaire was used in their research. Similarly, Nehring (1990) replicated earlier studies by Knox and Mogan (1985) and Mogan and Knox (1987) including the use of the NCTEI. Pugh (1988) has conducted a series of studies on clinical teaching effectiveness. This replication and extension of research reflects one of Pugh's (1983) recommendations from the earlier review of research.

CLINICAL TEACHING METHODS

This section of the review focuses on research on clinical teaching methods, such as patient assignment, conferences, and others. Clinical teaching methods are ways of organizing and presenting the instruction in the clinical setting to achieve learning outcomes (Reilly & Oermann, 1992). There were 46 studies on different clinical teaching methods including patient assignment ($n = 6$), written assignments ($n = 2$), clinical conference ($n = 5$), observation ($n = 2$), multimedia ($n = 16$), and preceptorships ($n = 15$).

Patient Assignment

Although patient assignment is the most widely used teaching method in the clinical setting, there are relatively few studies in this area. Early on, Kramer (1967) and Treece (1969) considered the process of selecting patients for student assignment and influence of student input into these assignments. Kramer's (1967) study was directed at identifying differences in the clinical experience when students ($n = 7$) chose their own assignment versus the instructor. Findings indicated that students have different clinical experiences when patient assignments are selected by the instructor than by themselves. The major limitation of the research, however, was the small sample size.

Treece (1969) surveyed 30 BSN students for their opinions about student selection of patients during clinical experiences. The majority of the sample (66.5%) indicated a desire for input into patient selection.

Glanville (1971) and Van Den Berg (1976) examined use of the multiple student assignment in clinical. Glanville (1971) randomly assigned 13 baccalaureate students to either a control or experimental group. The control group used a traditional assignment approach, one student per patient, while the experimental group used a multiple student assignment, a pair of students planning and delivering care to a patient, during a pediatric rotation. There were no significant differences between the groups in terms of knowledge and clinical performance. Lack of differences may be attributed to the small sample size, different clinical faculty, and differences in the clinical experiences of students through the course.

Van Den Berg (1976) randomly divided 22 first-year associate degree nursing students into two groups, traditional and multiple patient assignment. Students in the multiple student assignment group had the roles of doer, researcher, and observer. In the traditional group, each student was assigned at least one patient. Students in the multiple assignment group demonstrated significant improvement in nursing knowledge compared with the other group. Even though Van Den Berg used a random sampling technique, the small sample size limits generalizability.

McCoin and Jenkins (1988) identified five methods of preplanning activities for clinical experiences. Using a survey design, an open-ended instrument was completed by second year nursing students ($n = 34$) and faculty ($n = 46$) randomly selected from ADN programs in Tennessee. Validity and reliability of the questionnaire were not reported by the investigators. Faculty reported using the instructor assigned/student gathered method most frequently in which the teacher assigns a particular patient to the student, and the student then gathers information about the client. Replication of the research in other ADN programs and at the BSN level would provide a better understanding of how assignments are made for students and impact on learning outcomes.

In terms of preparing for psychiatric clinical experiences, Nieswiadomy, Arnold, and Johnson (1989) investigated whether or not students, in one

BSN program, should be assigned to read the client's chart before caring for patients. An experimental design was used in which students were randomly assigned into the experimental and control groups. Anxiety was measured by the State-Trait Anxiety Inventory (STAI) developed by Spielberger, Gorsuch, and Lushene (1970). Alpha coefficients ranged from .83 to .92 for the state scale and .86 to .92 for the trait scale. There were no significant differences in anxiety between students ($n = 58$) who read the patient's chart and a second group of students ($n = 60$) who did not read the chart prior to the first interaction with the client. The researchers concluded that for most students reading or not reading the patient's records does not significantly affect anxiety.

Research is needed to guide clinical faculty in decisions on patients to assign considering the outcomes of the experience and needs, interests, and characteristics of the student. Differences in patient assignment across types of clinical settings, for instance tertiary care, homes, and community sites, and the nature of the experience with individual patients and families should be examined through research.

Written Assignments

Written assignments which accompany the clinical experience may be effective strategies for organizing thinking, promoting development of critical thinking skills, and enhancing understanding of content (Allen, Bowers, & Diekelmann, 1989; Berg & Serenko, 1993; Reilly & Oermann, 1992). Considering the quantity of written assignments students complete in many nursing programs, however, research is limited as to their effectiveness.

An early study compared two charting methods for use as a teaching tool (Mitchell & Atwood, 1975). No significant differences were found between problem-oriented charting and traditional charting methods when evaluating case studies.

More recently, Sedlak (1992) examined the use of clinical logs for beginning nursing students. Twenty sophomore nursing students wrote in a weekly log their reactions to clinical experiences. Descriptive analyses identified major themes including learning from their own mistakes and negative experiences, self-growth in caring for complex patients, greater awareness of own emotions, recognition of improved communication skills, examination of own motivation, and awareness of ability to teach clients. Sedlak (1992) concluded that clinical logs provide an opportunity for self-reflection, facilitate communication with the teacher, involve the students actively in learning, and promote identification of own motivation as a learner.

In many nursing programs, written assignments are predominant clinical teaching methods; research on the outcomes and benefits to students, however, is lacking. The value of assignments such as care plans in promoting critical thinking and problem solving has not been established in the research. Meyers (1986) suggests that written assignments for critical thinking should be short analytical papers which give students an opportunity to puzzle over issues and formulate their own independent judgments. Research is needed on the outcomes and benefits of different written assignments for clinical.

Clinical Conferences

O'Shea (1970) concluded that neither post conference nor independent study guides were a superior method of post clinical study. In this two-year study with ADN students ($n = 30$), there were no differences in their performance on tests based on the use of study guides and post clinical conferences. A large percentage of students considered both methods to be helpful to their learning.

In three studies on clinical conferences (Craig & Page, 1981; Scholdra & Quiring, 1973; Wang & Blumberg, 1983), findings suggested that low-level questions were the predominant type asked by the teacher during interactions with learners. Sixteen instructors, and students in their clinical groups, participated in Scholdra and Quiring's (1973) early research on the level of questions posed by faculty. The investigators taped and analyzed 22 clinical conferences averaging 63 minutes each, categorizing the questions asked by the teacher. The pattern of questioning which teachers used in conferences included predominantly lower level questions even when the objectives reflected higher level outcomes. Lower level questions reflected 98.9% of the total number of questions asked by teachers and students.

Craig and Page (1981) randomly assigned instructors ($n = 14$) to an experimental group, which completed a self-instructional module on how to ask high-level questions during an interaction, and a control group. The dependent variable was the number of higher level questions asked by the instructor during a 30-minute recorded segment of a post clinical conference. The independent variable was the instructional module on questioning. The module was found to have a significant effect on the level of questions asked during post conference. The researchers concluded that faculty could improve their questioning skills.

Wang and Blumberg (1983) made 44 two-hour observations of clinical faculty in the field and recorded the frequency of 16 interaction techniques. One-third of the interactions between student and teacher lasted one minute or less; another third lasted one to six minutes. The majority of student-faculty interactions were on a one-to-one basis. Techniques used most frequently were leading and directing questions or information giving. Low-level questions, involving factual and procedural information, were asked most frequently.

Similar to the earlier study by Craig and Page (1981), Wink (1993a) found that faculty could develop ability to ask higher-level questions by completing an educational program in this area. She examined the effect of a program to increase the percentage of high-level questions asked in post conference; high-level questions assist students in applying knowledge to new and unique clinical situations (Wink, 1993b). Fourteen faculty and students in their clinical groups participated in the research. Pre- and posttest data were collected on the cognitive level of questions asked in conference for both the treatment ($n = 10$) and control ($n = 4$) groups using audiotapes. The treatment group completed a program designed to increase the level of questions asked by clinical faculty during post conference. There was no significant difference between the groups prior to the intervention. After completing the educational program, however, faculty in the treatment group increased the cognitive level of their questions ($U = 4$, $p = .012$). Because of the small sample size, the findings should be interpreted with caution; replication is needed with larger samples and in varied settings.

Considering the extent of questioning and discussion within the context of patient care and in conferences, research in this area is critical. One theme across studies is the low leveling of questioning by teachers focusing on recall and memorization of information rather than higher level questions stimulating analytical thinking, judgments, and evaluations of client care and decisions. Two studies demonstrated higher level questions posed by faculty who had attended an educational program.

Observation

Only a few early studies are available on the effects of student observation of experiences in the clinical setting (Embury & Thurston, 1976; Schulman, Foley, & Voorsanger, 1966). Weak study designs and questionable outcome measures combined with the limited number of studies make it difficult to draw conclusions about using observation in the clinical setting as a teaching method. Questions remain as to the outcomes and benefits to the learner of observing others in the clinical field prior to own performance.

Multimedia

There is a large body of research in nursing education on the effectiveness of multimedia, although fewer studies focus on using media for clinical teaching. Oermann (1990) concluded from a review of research on multimedia that media was as effective as other teaching methods in assisting students to acquire knowledge relevant to clinical practice and develop beginning practice skills. In some of the research comparing the effectiveness of media to lecture, clinical performance was included as a dependent variable (Arnold, 1978; Friesen & Stotts, 1984; Koniak, 1985; Stein, Steele, Fuller, & Langhoff, 1972; Sullivan & Weber, 1970). Findings indicated that media was at least as effective as lecture and lecture-discussion in terms of improving performance.

A few studies are available on teaching psychomotor skills with varying media and settings. Baldwin, Hill, and Hanson (1991) compared two teaching strategies, textbook assignment and videotaping with no faculty assistance and textbook assignment and videotaping with faculty guidance, to determine the effect on taking a blood pressure. Seventeen baccalaureate students were randomly assigned to these two groups. A significant difference was found between the groups. The researchers suggested that while videotaping may be used for learning skills, faculty contact during the instruction was important.

Videotaping was also examined in earlier research to teach interviewing to nurse practitioner students (Sullivan, Grover, Lynaugh, & Levy, 1975); improve clinical observation skills (Jeffers & Christensen, 1979); and enhance clinical performance and participation in post clinical conferences (Griffin, Kinsinger, Pitman, & Kessler, 1966). Videotaping was found to be of value in promoting the development of selected practice skills such as interviewing.

In terms of computer-assisted instruction (CAI), the majority of research focuses on the use of CAI for learning theoretical content or instruction in a learning laboratory. Studies have been done, however, comparing computer simulation to role play for learning interviewing techniques (Droste-Bielak, 1986); evaluating students' decision-making skills by computer simulations (Lowdermilk & Fishel, 1991; Wong, Wong, & Richard, 1994); using interactive video to simulate clinical practice (Fishman, 1984; Rickelman, Taylor-Fox, Reisch, Payne, & Jelemensky, 1988); and comparing the effectiveness of CAI and small-group review for teaching clinical calculations, such as calculating drug dosages (Gilbert & Kolacz, 1993). The intent of this review is not to critique research on CAI but instead to indicate that some research has been done exploring the effect of CAI on clinical knowledge and performance.

In one other study involving computers, Howse, Smith, and Perkin (1994) developed a computer system for assigning students to clinical settings and compared this method with assigning students by hand. In the latter traditional method, students identified their first three choices for clinical placement and were then assigned an agency based on their preferences, faculty input, and nature and number of available settings.

The assignor attempted to match the student's abilities with the demands of the clinical setting. For the development of the computer program, student preferences were factored into the program to avoid placing students in their least-desired setting. Criteria for matching students and setting were established. The assignment by computer was found to be more accurate and efficient, in terms of time, than assigning students by hand.

The studies on media and CAI which have used clinical performance as an outcome measure suggest that these teaching methods are appropriate for developing clinical skills. Further research should examine the interaction of different learner characteristics and use of multimedia and effect of these on outcomes of learning.

Preceptorships

There are increasing numbers of studies on preceptorships in nursing programs. Findings of the research suggest benefits for students including (1) improved socialization, (2) transition to the staff nurse role, (3) improved clinical competence and performance, and (4) increased self-confidence (Clayton, Broome, & Ellis, 1989; Collins, Hilde, & Shriver, 1993; Dobbs, 1988; Hughes, Wade, & Peters, 1991; Jairath, Costello, Wallace, & Rudy, 1991; Koehler, Broome, Clayton, & Morse, 1988; Myrick & Awrey, 1988; Oermann & Navin, 1991; Scheetz, 1989; Yonge & Trojan, 1992). Benefits for the preceptors themselves, such as keeping them challenged and stimulated, also have been reported (Bizek & Oermann, 1990).

Two of the first studies focused on the role conceptions and role deprivation of students participating in a preceptorship. In Itano, Warren, and Ishida's (1987) research, 118 BSN students completed the Corwin Nursing Role Conception tool. Content validity and reliability of this instrument were established in other studies. No differences were found in role conceptions or role deprivation between students who participated in a preceptor program and traditional faculty supervised clinical experience.

Dobbs (1988) measured anticipatory socialization among BSN students ($n = 103$) following a preceptorship experience. Students completed Corwin's instrument before and after a final clinical course which was preceptor-based. Paired t-tests indicated a significant decrease in role deprivation and significant increase in number of work-centered role models. Lack of a control group, however, limits the value of the findings.

Other studies have examined the performance of students following a preceptorship as the outcome variable. Myrick and Awrey (1988) compared seven preceptored and five nonpreceptored nursing students using Schwirian's (1978) Six-Dimension (6-D) Scale of Nursing Performance. The 6-D Scale is composed of 52 items grouped into six performance categories: leadership, critical care, teaching/collaboration, planning/evaluation, interpersonal relations, and professional development. Cronbach's alpha ranged from .84 to .98 for the subscales. Students who were supervised by a preceptor had a more positive view of their performance than the nonpreceptored group and engaged in more planning and evaluative behaviors, although results must be interpreted with caution considering the small sample size.

Clayton et al. (1989) studied the relationship between a preceptorship experience and role socialization of graduate nurses. A quasi-experimental design was used with two groups of BSN students in their final clinical course. In the experimental group, students ($n = 33$) were paired one-to-one with a preceptor. Students in the control group ($n = 33$) had a traditional course under the direction of a clinical faculty. Schwirian's (1978) 6-D Scale was administered at three testing points, prior to the course, immediately following the course, and six months after graduation. The group with the preceptorship experience scored higher on five of the six subscales of the instrument at the end of the course. At the six-month follow-up, the preceptor group scored higher on four of the subscales. The researchers concluded that working with a preceptor eased transition into the staff nurse role.

Scheetz (1989) reported that students who completed a preceptor experience ($n = 36$) had significantly greater gains in clinical competency than students who worked as nursing assistants ($n = 36$). Using a non-equivalent comparison group pretest-posttest design, Scheetz examined students' clinical competence and other variables following a summer preceptorship and non-instructional work experience. Competence was measured by the Clinical Competence Rating Scale (CCRS) which consists of 53 nursing behaviors on problem-solving ability, application of theory to practice, and psychomotor skill. Interrater reliability ranged from .80 to .86 for the total CCRS, although some of the subscales were higher; the alpha coefficient was .96 to .97. Analysis of covariance indicated that students who completed the summer preceptor experience gained greater levels of clinical competence than students who worked as nursing assistants. Both groups of subjects, however, reported that their experiences enabled them to develop problem-solving skills, apply theory to practice, improve their psychomotor skills, and develop more self-confidence in their nursing role. Scheetz (1989) found no significant correlation between grade point average (GPA) and clinical competence and no significant differences between the groups in terms of age, GPA, prior work or volunteer experience in health care settings, and other variables which might potentially influence ratings of clinical competence. Control of these variables is an important need in the research.

Hsieh and Knowles (1990), identified seven themes important in developing an effective relationship with the preceptor using naturalistic observations and feedback from 12 preceptors, 12 students, and two instructors. These themes were trust; clearly defined expectations; support systems for preceptors, students, and instructor support for both; honest communication; mutual respect and acceptance; encouragement; and mutual sharing of self and experience. Development of these themes early in the preceptor-student relationship facilitated progress toward achieving the learning objectives of the preceptorship.

Using a quasi-experimental design, Jairath, Costello, Wallace, and Rudy (1991), examined the effect of a 17-week preceptor experience upon diploma nursing students' ($n = 22$) performance. Subjects were enrolled in the final semester of a three-year diploma program at a community college in Canada. Nine students participated in the preceptor experience; the remaining 13 completed the traditional clinical course. Similar to a number of other studies, the 6-D Scale was used to measure performance; the instrument was administered prior to, during, and at the completion of the preceptorship. There were no differences in performance at 4 weeks. At 17 weeks, however, the experimental group had significantly greater increases in teaching/collaboration and planning/evaluation. Both groups improved significantly in all areas of performance except for leadership. From the students' perspective, working with a preceptor was not associated with greater increases in performance over time. Once again the small sample size, particularly in the preceptor group, limits drawing conclusions about the preceptorship experience.

Pierce (1991) approached the study of preceptorship from a different point of view, that of the student. In this qualitative study, 29 first- and 15 second-level undergraduate students described outcomes they desired from the preceptorship. The research built on an earlier study by Windsor (1987) using similar questions. Outcomes desired by students included, an opportunity to care for a range of patients and a chance to try new skills. An important requirement from the student's perspective was an interested preceptor who had expertise as a clinician and teacher. Pierce (1991) emphasized that faculty need to provide clear directives about the intended clinical learning experiences and objectives of the course, provide support to preceptors and others in the clinical setting, and follow up on the clinical experiences to assure that the outcomes are achieved.

Yonge and Trojan (1992) compared the performance of preceptored ($n = 38$) and nonpreceptored ($n = 33$) students, although a complete data set was obtained for only 9 students in the preceptor group and 19 in the nonpreceptored group. Students rated their performance pre- and post clinical using the 6-D Scale. Instructors and preceptors rated students at the end of the clinical rotation. ANOVA for repeated measures indicated that both groups of students changed in these six dimensions from pre- to post clinical. Nonpreceptored students had significantly higher scores than preceptored students in all areas except critical care. The small sample size and differences in the size of the groups limit conclusions which may be drawn from the findings.

Although preceptorships have become a recognized clinical teaching method, only one study has examined criteria for selecting preceptors. At times preceptors are selected primarily because of their availability (Myrick & Barrett, 1994). Myrick and Barrett (1992) surveyed baccalaureate schools of nursing in Canada to determine the criteria used for the selection of clinical preceptors. Twenty-five programs were represented. While most (70%) schools used preceptors for clinical teaching, typically in the last year of the nursing program, only 45% defined specific criteria for their selection. The major criteria used to select clinical preceptors included clinical competence, commitment to the preceptor role, effective communication skills, skilled use of the nursing process, and professional conduct.

Summary

While there is variability in the quality of research on preceptorship experiences for students and outcomes evaluated, the findings suggest benefits for students of such experiences. Considering the studies as a whole, working with a preceptor as a student appears to ease the transition to the role of the nurse, improve performance, and increase self-confidence. Whether a preceptored experience is better than a traditional faculty directed practicum or other concentrated clinical experience in terms of performance, role development, and self-confidence has not yet been established in the research.

Research on preceptorships needs to be extended and longitudinal in nature to examine if these benefits continue over time and identify variables which are essential for an effective preceptor experience. It is critical for larger samples to be used, and for researchers to control or at least account for factors which might influence the effectiveness of such experiences, such as prior work experience of the student. Other questions to be answered relate to the criteria used for selecting preceptors; effect of preceptor characteristics such as educational level, prior experience as a preceptor, and preparation for carrying out the preceptor role; and process of evaluating their effectiveness in the clinical setting. This is an area of research in which replications of studies would contribute to our understanding of the outcomes of preceptor experiences and how they should be designed for students.

STUDENT PERCEPTIONS OF CLINICAL

The third area of research on clinical teaching relates to the student and his or her experience in clinical practice. Studies in this area deal with student stress and anxiety in the clinical setting, student perceptions of their clinical experience, and effects of clinical on student development of self-concept. Ten studies were reviewed predominantly on student stress in clinical.

Student Stress in Clinical

Research on the stress experienced by students in clinical practice is emerging. Pagana (1988) identified the stresses and threats reported by students ($n = 262$) in their first clinical experience in medical-surgical nursing. The degrees of stress and challenge were measured by the Clinical Stress Questionnaire (CSQ) developed by the investigator. Factor analysis supported the construct validity of the CSQ. The alpha coefficients were between .84 and .85, and inter-rater reliability for the open-ended responses was .89 (Pagana, 1989). The mean stress score was 2.7 on a scale of 0 (none at all) to 4 (a great deal). Students were significantly more challenged than threatened in this initial experience particularly by the opportunity to apply knowledge and skills in clinical. Six major threats were reported: feelings of personal inadequacy, fear of making errors, uncertainty, fear of the clinical instructor, being frightened, and fear of failure. The majority of subjects ($n = 202$, 77.1%) described feelings of personal inadequacy; eighty-nine (34%) feared they would harm the patient by making an error. Sixty-eight (26%) subjects perceived the clinical instructor as a threat. Pearson correlation coefficient revealed significant relationships between stress and feelings of inadequacy (r = .28, $p < .001$), fear of failure (r = .24, $p < .001$), and being frightened (r = .22, $p < .001$). The higher the stress level, the more likely were these threats. Pagana (1989) reported on the psychometric evaluation of the CSQ used in this research.

In a related study, Pagana (1990) examined the relationship of hardiness and social support to student appraisal of stress. There was a significant positive correlation, although weak, between challenge and hardiness (r = .23, $p < .001$). Subjects who were less hardy had higher threat scores although the correlation was low. No significant relationship was found between total functional social support and challenge, except the scale that refers to network members helping one relax after a clinical experience (Pagana, 1990). This correlation, however, also was low.

Similarly, Kleehammer, Hart, and Keck (1990) reported that students were most anxious during the initial clinical experience on the unit and had the greatest fear of making a mistake. A convenience sample of 39 junior and 53 senior baccalaureate nursing students from one BSN program completed the Clinical Experience Assessment Form. The 16 items on the Likert scale instrument addressed communication, procedural aspects of care, interpersonal relationships with health care providers, and interactions with faculty. Cronbach's alpha was .82; factor analysis established construct validity.

Aspects of care such as talking to patients, providing morning care, and patient teaching were not anxiety producing for these students. Higher levels of anxiety, however, included the initial clinical experience on a unit and fear of making mistakes, similar to findings of other studies (Kushnir, 1986; Pagana, 1988; Williams, 1993). Performing procedures, talking with physicians, and being observed and evaluated by faculty created anxiety for them. The qualitative data suggested that student perceptions of nonsupportive faculty increased their anxiety in the clinical setting.

In research by Beck and Srivastava (1991) involved 94 BSN students. Stressful events identified by students included lacking clinical knowledge and experience for practice ($n = 16$) and a combination of unfamiliarity in the clinical field and difficult patients ($n = 14$). Developing relationships with patients, engaging in new learning experiences, and helping others were ranked highest as areas of satisfaction.

In Williams' (1993) study of concerns of beginning nursing students, once again this fear of harming the patient was reported. The sample included 245 beginning nursing students across five campuses. The instrument, developed by the investigator, included 38 items on a Likert scale. The instrument had content validity and an alpha coefficient of .93. The greatest concerns to these students were keeping up with their grades, fear of doing something wrong to the patient, and learning clinical procedures. These latter two concerns regarding clinical practice were expressed by the majority of respondents.

Similar to this research, Reider and Riley-Giomariso (1993) found that students experienced anxiety in the initial clinical experience associated with a nursing leadership course. This anticipatory anxiety included stress related to non-specific concerns including fear of the unknown; communication with nursing staff, physicians and others; and carrying out and managing nursing functions. Using a qualitative design, Reider and Riley-Giomariso (1993) collected data from 27 senior baccalaureate nursing students enrolled in a leadership course. Subjects were interviewed and completed logs during their experience. Other themes reflected outcomes of a leadership experience, including opportunity to clarify the leadership role in nursing, develop leadership skills and self-confidence, and gain entrance into the nursing delivery system.

Qualitative Studies on Student Perceptions of Clinical

Windsor (1987) interviewed nine senior nursing students to describe this experience from the learner's point of view in a qualitative study on students' perceptions of their clinical experience. Major categories of learning included practice of nursing skills, time management, and professional socialization through observing nurses in practice. The data also suggested that students progressed through three stages of development. In the first stage, students were anxious about clinical and oriented toward nursing tasks. The second stage involved a transition into the role of the professional nurse. In the last stage, students were more confident and independent in practice.

In another qualitative study, Wilson (1994) explored the student's clinical experience with acutely ill infants. Data were collected through observations of students in a pediatric setting for approximately 75 hours over two semesters. Observations were made of students providing care to patients and their interactions with others. Interviews were conducted with 30 students within one day following the observation period. Six major goals of the clinical experience emerged from the study: avoid harming the patient, help the patient, integrate theory into practice, develop clinical skills, and "look good" both as a student and nurse.

Student Self-Concept

A number of studies, described earlier in the review, examined the effects of preceptor experiences on professional socialization and role development of students. In addition to these, Hughes, Wade, and Peters (1991) reported on the effects of a synthesis course on senior baccalaureate nursing students' ($n = 70$) self-concept and role competencies. Self-concept was measured by the Tennessee Self-Concept Scale; the Slater Nursing Competency Scale was used to measure subjects' perceptions of role competencies. A one-group pretest-posttest design was used for the research. There was a significant increase in students' self-concept and their perceptions of role competencies upon completion of the course.

A more comprehensive evaluation of factors affecting student competency and development of self-confidence was completed by Mozingo, Thomas, and Brooks (1995). In this study involving 204 BSN students from one program, both quantitative and qualitative data were collected using multiple instruments: STAI, Norbeck's Social Support Questionnaire, and Perceived Competency Scale developed by the investigators. This latter instrument consisted of 12 items on perceived clinical competence on a Likert scale. The alpha coefficient was .83. Completion of an externship did not influence perceived clinical competency. Pearson r indicated a significant relationship between employment in a health care setting during the nursing program and competency ($r = .26$, $p = .0001$). There was an inverse relationship between anxiety and competency ($r = -.31$, $p = .0001$). Students reported lack of competency with technical skills. The research builds on other studies which measure particular outcomes of clinical and needs to be replicated with other groups of students.

Summary

While research is beginning to document the stresses and threats experienced by students in clinical practice and their perceptions of the clinical experience, more study is indicated in this area. Differences in stress across types of nursing programs, clinical courses and settings, levels of students, and types of clinical experiences need further investigation. Research in this area should be replicated in other BSN programs and in ADN and graduate programs in which research is lacking. Student characteristics that influence their perceptions of stressful events in clinical practice and the degree of stress experienced have yet to be determined through research.

CLINICAL EXPERIENCE IN GENERAL

The last theme of research on clinical teaching has examined the clinical experience in general. Studies in this category do not relate to the clinical teacher, teaching methods, or student perceptions. Instead, the research deals with the effects of different types of clinical experiences and courses and how to design them. Eleven studies were reviewed in this section.

Structure of Clinical Practicum

Porter and Feller (1979) failed to demonstrate that students in practicums which extended over a longer period of time had increased knowledge and self-confidence in comparison with ones lasting fewer weeks. They examined the effect of the pattern of clinical experience on achievement among 91 generic BSN students and 10 nursing faculty. Students and faculty were randomly assigned to either distributive clinical time involving clinical practice over 16 weeks, eight hours per week in one setting and eight hours in a second practice site. The massed clinical time group had a concentration of clinical time in one setting for eight weeks followed by a concentrated time in the second setting for another eight weeks. There were no significant differences in student achievement as measured by NLN Achievement Tests in Medical-Surgical Nursing and Community Health Nursing, state board scores, and scores on two simulations which focused on application of knowledge.

More recently, Dunn, Stockhausen, Thornton, and Barnard (1995) examined the relationship between the clinical education format, reflecting the structure, organization, and timing of the clinical practicum, and selected student outcomes in a BSN program in Australia. Both quantitative and qualitative data were collected. A convenience sample of 64 students was assigned to one of two formats, one day/week of clinical practice or two consecutive days once every two weeks. Neither was found to be more effective across the different learning outcomes.

In a different line of research, Infante tested her clinical teaching model with 173 baccalaureate students randomly assigned to experimental and control groups (Infante, Forbes, Houldin, & Naylor, 1989). In the experimental group, the clinical experience emphasized use of the learning laboratory, integrated theory and clinical practice, and provided for student participation in clinical, among other features. Students in the experimental group had higher grade point averages, higher scores on the Mosby Assesstest, and higher practicum scores than the control group.

Course-Specific Experiences

Another area of research has focused on the types of clinical experiences provided students in particular courses and the curriculum as a whole. This type of research includes studies by Alley, Doneckers, and King (1992) on the clinical practicum in graduate programs in home health care; by McEwen (1992) on community health nursing clinical experiences in baccalaureate programs; and on the effects of particular clinical experiences such as caring for disabled patients (Lindgren & Oermann, 1993; Oermann & Lindgren, 1995), experiences with the elderly (Dellasega & Curriero, 1991; Hartley, Bentz, & Ellis, 1995; Reinhardy & Quam, 1989), and clinical practice sites for students in psychiatric nursing courses (Slimmer, Wendt, & Martinkus, 1990).

Summary

Research in this last section is varied, but points to the need for study on the organization of the clinical practicum and effectiveness of different types of clinical courses within the curriculum.

CONCLUSIONS AND RECOMMENDATIONS

The research on clinical teaching focuses predominantly on the teacher and behaviors reflecting clinical teaching effectiveness. Some generalizations were drawn from this research suggesting characteristics of an effective clinical teacher although further studies are indicated with larger and more diverse samples. Measurements of clinical teacher effectiveness over time, for instance, at the beginning and end of the semester, have not been reported in the literature and would add an important dimension to this research. A related question is whether student perceptions of teacher effectiveness vary over time. Few of the studies have examined the influence of the type of clinical course, clinical setting, level of student, and teacher variables, such as the extent of teaching and clinical experience, on ratings of teacher effectiveness. Differences, if any, in student perceptions of teaching effectiveness between full- and part-time faculty and whether the clinical teacher is an instructor from the nursing program or a clinician from the health care agency have not been examined in this research.

There is limited research to guide faculty in making decisions as to patients to select for learners and other clinical experiences. The effectiveness of various written assignments associated with the clinical experience, such as nursing care plans, has not been established through research. There is an emerging body of nursing literature on critical thinking and the formation of clinical judgments essential for care of clients. Research is needed on clinical experiences and teaching methods which most effectively encourage development of these cognitive skills among learners. The use of multimedia, particularly interactive video; impact on clinical decision making and judgment in the clinical setting; and relationship to other experiences in the clinical setting need investigation. It is clear even from the limited research available that faculty ask low-level questions, requiring recall and memorization rather than evaluation and judgment, of students in the clinical field and in conferences. These higher level questions, however, are important to promote critical thinking in the practice setting (Reilly & Oermann, 1992). Faculty development programs may be indicated to raise the level of questions asked of learners; research, although limited, suggests that instructional programs may be of value in assisting faculty to improve their questioning skills.

While research is available on preceptorships, studies need to be replicated with other groups of students and preceptors and in different settings and areas of the country. Much of the research involves small sample sizes and has been conducted in one setting only, limiting generalizability. Another problem in terms of generalizing the results is that varying outcome measures have been used to examine the effects of preceptor programs. Criteria for selecting preceptors; differences across levels of students, courses, and programs; educational programs to prepare preceptors for clinical teaching; and evaluations conducted of their clinical teaching effectiveness are areas needing further study. The effects of preceptor experiences over time also need to be studied. Baird, Bopp, Schofer, Langenberg, and Matheis-Kraft (1994) and Melander and Roberts (1994) describe the use of clinical teaching associates to assist faculty in the direct supervision of students. As other models of clinical teaching emerge, such as this one, research is needed on their effectiveness. Similarly, as clinical experiences continue to shift into the community and newer settings, research needs to examine the outcomes of these experiences and provide guidance to faculty who are teaching in these sites.

Few studies identify characteristics of the learner and teacher and their relationship to the clinical experience and methods of teaching used in the clinical setting. The individual teacher may exert a major influence on the outcomes of clinical. Few researchers attempt to account for the influence of the teacher, and in some studies the preceptor, on outcomes measured. There are many anecdotal reports in the literature on strategies for teaching in the clinical setting and benefits of different clinical experiences for students; research is needed, however, to substantiate the apparent benefits of these experiences.

As seen in other nursing research, there is a lack of replication of studies in the setting of the original research and with different populations. With many studies on clinical teaching, larger samples are indicated. The majority of studies focus on some aspect of baccalaureate nursing education; research should be extended to other types of nursing programs. There is scattered research with ADN students; clinical teaching in graduate programs has not been studied. Few nurse educators have extended their work, except for some researchers on teacher effectiveness, and one-time studies dominate. The need remains for further study on clinical teaching and the clinical experience in general to continue to establish a theoretical and research base for teaching students in the clinical setting.

REFERENCES

Allen, D. G., Bowers, B., & Diekelmann, N. (1989). Writing to learn: A reconceptualization of thinking and writing in the nursing curriculum. *Journal of Nursing Education, 28,* 6–11.

Alley, J. M., Doneckers, S. W., & King, J. C. (1992). Integrating experienced and novice nurses into graduate home health education. *Journal of Nursing Education, 31,* 357–360.

Armington, C. L., Reinikka, E. A., & Creighton, H. (1972). Student evaluation: Threat or incentive. *Nursing Outlook, 20,* 789–792.

Arnold, J. (1978). Let's discuss teaching strategies. *Journal of Nursing Education, 17,* 15–20.

Baird, S. C., Bopp, A., Schofer, K. K., Langenberg, A. S., & Matheis-Kraft, C. (1994). An innovative model for clinical teaching. *Nurse Educator, 19*(3), 23–25.

Baldwin, D., Hill, P., & Hanson, G. (1991). Performance of psychomotor skills: A comparison of two teaching strategies. *Journal of Nursing Education, 30,* 367–370.

Barham, V. (1965). Identifying effective behavior of the nursing instructor through critical incidents. *Nursing Research, 14,* 65–69.

Beck, C. T. (1991). How students perceive faculty caring: A phenomenological study. *Nurse Educator, 16*(5), 18–22.

Beck, D. L., & Srivastava, R. (1990). Perceived level and sources of stress in baccalaureate nursing students. *Journal of Nursing Education, 30,* 127–133.

Berg, J., & Serenko, P. C. (1993). Teaching professional writing skills to the baccalaureate student. *Journal of Nursing Education, 32,* 329.

Bergman, K., & Gaitskill, T. (1990). Faculty and student perceptions of effective clinical teachers: An extension study. *Journal of Professional Nursing, 6*(1), 33–44.

Bizek, K. S., & Oermann, M. H. (1991). Study of educational experiences, support, and job satisfaction among critical care preceptors. *Heart & Lung, 19,* 439–444.

Brown, S. T. (1981). Faculty and student perceptions of effective clinical teachers. *Journal of Nursing Education, 20,* 4–15.

Clayton, G. M., Broome, M. E., & Ellis, L. A. (1989). Relationship between a preceptorship experience and role socialization of graduate nurses. *Journal of Nursing Education, 28,* 72–75.

Collins, P., Hilde, E., & Shriver, C. (1993). A five-year evaluation of BSN students in a nursing management preceptorship. *Journal of Nursing Education, 32,* 330–332.

Craig, J. L., & Page, G. (1981). The questioning skills of nursing instructors. *Journal of Nursing Education, 20,* 18–23.

Dellasega, C., & Curriero, F. C. (1991). The effects of institutional and community experiences on nursing students' intentions toward work with the elderly. *Journal of Nursing Education, 30,* 405–410.

de Tornyay, R. (1993). Nursing education: Staying on track. *Nursing & Health Care, 14,* 302–306.

Dobbs, K. K. (1988). The senior preceptorship as a method of anticipatory socialization of baccalaureate nursing students. *Journal of Nursing Education, 27,* 167–171.

Droste-Bielak, E. M. (1986). Two techniques for teaching interviewing: A comparative study. *Computers in Nursing, 4,* 152–157.

Dunn, S. V., Stockhausen, L., Thornton, R., & Barnard, A. (1995). The relationship between clinical education format and selected student learning outcomes. *Journal of Nursing Education, 34,* 16–23.

Embury, S. B., & Thurston, N. B. (1976). A preliminary study on the effect of role modeling on anxiety in motor skill performance and the effect of self concept on motor skill performance. *Nursing Papers, 8*(3), 33–39.

Fishman, D. J. (1984). Development and evaluation of a computer assisted video module for teaching cancer chemotherapy to nurses. *Computers in Nursing, 2,* 16–23.

Flagler, S., Loper-Powers, S., & Spitzer, A. (1988). Clinical teaching is more than evaluation alone! *Journal of Nursing Education, 27,* 342–348.

Fong, C. M., & McCauley, G. T. (1993). Measuring the nursing, teaching, and interpersonal effectiveness of clinical instructors. *Journal of Nursing Education, 32,* 325–328.

Friesen, L., & Stotts, N. A. (1984). Retention of basic cardiac life support content: The effect of two teaching methods. *Journal of Nursing Education, 27,* 30–34.

Gilbert, D. A., & Kolacz, N. G. (1993). Effectiveness of CAI and small-group review in teaching clinical calculation. *Computers in Nursing, 11,* 72–77.

Glanville, C. L. (1971). Multiple student assignments as an approach to clinical teaching in pediatric nursing. *Nursing Research, 20,* 237–244.

Griffin, G. J., Kinsinger, R. E., Pitman, A. J., & Kessler, E. R. (1966). New dimensions for the improvement of clinical nursing. *Nursing Research, 15,* 292–302.

Hartley, C. L., Bentz, P. M., & Ellis, J. R. (1995). The effect of early nursing home placement on student attitudes toward the elderly. *Journal of Nursing Education, 34,* 128–130.

Horst, M. E. (1988). Students rank characteristics of the clinical teacher. *Nurse Educator, 13*(6), 3.

Howse, E., Smith, B., & Perkin, C. A. (1994). Differences between manual and computer-based methods for clinical learning assignments. *Computers in Nursing, 12,* 280–288.

Hsieh, N. L., & Knowles, D. W. (1990). Instructor facilitation of the preceptorship relationship in nursing education. *Journal of Nursing Education, 29,* 262–268.

Hughes, O., Wade, B., & Peters, M. (1991). The effects of a synthesis of nursing practice course on senior nursing students' self-concept and role perception. *Journal of Nursing Education, 30,* 69–72.

Infante, M. S., Forbes, E. J., Houldin, A. D., & Naylor, M. (1989). A clinical teaching project: Examination of a clinical teaching model. *Journal of Professional Nursing, 5*, 132–139.

Itano, J. K., Warren, J. J., & Ishida, D. N. (1987). A comparison of role conceptions and role deprivation of baccalaureate students in nursing participating in a preceptorship or a traditional clinical program. *Journal of Nursing Education, 26*, 69–73.

Jacobson, M. D. (1966). Effective and ineffective behavior of teachers of nursing as determined by their students. *Nursing Research, 15*, 218–224.

Jairath, N., Costello, J., Wallace, P., & Rudy, L. (1991). The effect of preceptorship upon diploma program nursing students' transition to the professional nursing role. *Journal of Nursing Education, 30*, 251–255.

Jeffers, J. M., & Christensen, M. G. (1979). Using simulation to facilitate the acquisition of clinical observational skills. *Journal of Nursing Education, 18*(6), 29–32.

Karns, P. J., & Schwab, T. A. (1982). Therapeutic communication and clinical instruction. *Nursing Outlook, 30*, 39–43.

Kiker, M. (1973). Characteristics of the effective teacher. *Nursing Outlook, 21*, 721–723.

Kleehammer, K., Hart, A. L., & Keck, J. F. (1990). Nursing students' perceptions of anxiety-producing situations in the clinical setting. *Journal of Nursing Education, 29*, 183–187.

Knox, J. E., & Mogan, J. (1985). Important clinical teacher behaviours as perceived by university nursing faculty, students and graduates. *Journal of Advanced Nursing, 10*, 25–30.

Koehler, C., Broome, M., Clayton, G., & Morse, J. (1988). Rural preceptorship program for baccalaureate student. *Nurse Educator, 13*(2), 5–6.

Koniak, D. (1985). Autotutorial and lecture-demonstration instruction: A comparative analysis of the effects upon students' learning of a developmental assessment skill. *Western Journal of Nursing Research, 7*, 80–100.

Kramer, M. (1967). Does the teacher really know best? *Journal of Nursing Education, 6*(1), 3–24.

Kramer, M., Polifroni, E. C., & Organek, N. (1986). Effects of faculty practice on student learning outcomes. *Journal of Professional Nursing, 2*, 289–301.

Krichbaum, K. (1994). Clinical teaching effectiveness described in relation to learning outcomes of baccalaureate nursing students. *Journal of Nursing Education, 33*, 306–316.

Kushnir, T. (1986). Stress and social facilitation: The effects of the presence of an instructor on student nurses' behaviour. *Journal of Advanced Nursing, 11*, 13–19.

Lindgren, C. L., & Oermann, M. H. (1993). Effects of an educational intervention on students' attitudes toward the disabled. *Journal of Nursing Education, 32,* 121–126.

Lowdermilk, D. L., & Fishel, A. H. (1991). Computer simulations as a measure of nursing students' decision-making skills. *Journal of Nursing Education, 30,* 34–39.

McCoin, D. W., & Jenkins, P. C. (1988). Methods of assignment for preplanning activities (advance student preparation) for the clinical experience. *Journal of Nursing Education, 27,* 85–87.

McEwen, M. (1992). Community health nursing clinicals: An examination of the present and ideas for the future. *Journal of Nursing Education, 31,* 210–214.

Melander, S., & Roberts, C. (1994). Clinical teaching associate model: Creating effective BSN student/faculty/staff nurse triads. *Journal of Nursing Education, 33,* 422–425.

Meyers, C. (1986). *Teaching students to think critically.* San Francisco: Jossey-Bass.

Mims, F. (1970). Students evaluate faculty. *Nursing Outlook, 18,* 53–56.

Mitchell, P. H., & Atwood, J. (1975). Problem-oriented recording as a teaching-learning tool. *Nursing Research, 24,* 99–103.

Mogan, J., & Knox, J. E. (1987). Characteristics of 'best' and 'worst' clinical teachers as perceived by university nursing faculty and students. *Journal of Advanced Nursing, 12,* 331–337.

Mogan, J., & Warbinek, E. (1994). Teaching behaviours of clinical instructors: An audit instrument. *Journal of Advanced Nursing, 20,* 160–166.

Morgan, S. A. (1991). Teaching activities of clinical instructors during the direct client care period: A qualitative investigation. *Journal of Advanced Nursing, 16,* 1238–1246.

Mozingo, J., Thomas, S., & Brooks, E. (1995). Factors associated with perceived competency levels of graduating seniors in a baccalaureate program. *Journal of Nursing Education, 34,* 115–122.

Myrick, F., & Awrey, J. (1988). The effect of preceptorship on the clinical competency of baccalaureate student nurses: A pilot study. *Canadian Journal of Nursing Research, 20*(3), 29–43.

Myrick, F., & Barrett, C. (1992). Preceptor selection criteria in Canadian basic baccalaureate schools of nursing—a survey. *Canadian Journal of Nursing Research, 24*(3), 53–68.

Myrick, F., & Barrett, C. (1994). Selecting clinical preceptors for basic baccalaureate nursing students: A critical issue in clinical teaching. *Journal of Advanced Nursing, 19,* 194–198.

Nehring, V. (1990). Nursing clinical teacher effectiveness inventory: A replication study of characteristics of 'best' and 'worst' clinical teachers as perceived by nursing faculty and students. *Journal of Advanced Nursing, 15,* 934–940.

Nieswiadomy, R., Arnold, W. K., & Johnson, M. (1989). Chart reading and anxiety levels of nursing students prior to the first interactions with psychiatric clients. *Journal of Nursing Education, 28,* 67–71.

Oermann, M. H. (1990). Research on teaching methods. In G. M. Clayton & P. A. Baj (Eds.), *Review of research in nursing education* (Vol. III). New York: National League for Nursing Press.

Oermann, M. H. (1994a). Professional nursing education in the future: Changes and challenges. *Journal of Obstetric, Gynecologic, and Neonatal Nursing, 5*(1), 153–159.

Oermann, M. H. (1994b). Reforming nursing education for future practice. *Journal of Nursing Education, 33,* 215–219.

Oermann, M. H., & Lindgren, C. L. (1995). Effects of educational intervention on student attitudes toward disabled: One-year follow-up. *Rehabilitation Nursing, 20*(1).

Oermann, M. H., & Navin, M. A. (1991). Effect of extern experience on clinical competence of graduate nurses. *Nursing Connections, 4*(4), 2–9.

O'Shea, H. S. (1970). Reinforcing clinical study. *Nursing Outlook, 18*(7), 58–61.

O'Shea, H. S., & Parsons, M. K. (1979). Clinical instruction: Effective/ and ineffective teacher behaviors. *Nursing Outlook, 27,* 411–415.

Pagana, K. D. (1988). Stresses and threats reported by baccalaureate students in relation to an initial clinical experience. *Journal of Nursing Education, 27,* 418–424.

Pagana, K. D. (1989). Psychometric evaluation of the Clinical Stress Questionnaire (CSQ). *Journal of Nursing Education, 28,* 169–174.

Pagana, K. D. (1990). The relationship of hardiness and social support to student appraisal of stress in an initial clinical nursing situation. *Journal of Nursing Education, 29,* 255–261.

Pierce, A. G. (1991). Preceptorial students' view of their clinical experience. *Journal of Nursing Education, 30,* 244–250.

Piscopo, B. (1994). Organizational climate, communication, and role strain in clinical nursing faculty. *Journal of Professional Nursing, 10,* 113–119.

Porter, K., & Feller, C. (1979). The relationship between patterns of massed and distributive clinical practicum and student achievement. *Journal of Nursing Education, 18,* 27–34.

Pugh, E. J. (1983). Research on clinical teaching. In W. L. Holzemer (Ed.), *Review of research in nursing education* (pp. 62–77). Thorofare, NJ: Slack.

Pugh, E. J. (1988). Soliciting student input to improve clinical teaching. *Nurse Educator, 13*(5), 28–33.

Rauen, K. C. (1974). The clinical instructor as role model. *Journal of Nursing Education, 13,* 33–40.

Reeve, M. M. (1994). Development of an instrument to measure effectiveness of clinical instructors. *Journal of Nursing Education, 33,* 15–20.

Reider, J. A., & Riley-Giomariso, O. (1993). Baccalaureate nursing students' perspectives of their clinical nursing leadership experience. *Journal of Nursing Education, 32,* 127–132.

Reilly, D. E., & Oermann, M. H. (1992). *Clinical teaching in nursing education.* New York: National League for Nursing Press.

Reinhardy, J. R., & Quam, J. (1989). Providing health services to elderly in public housing: A case for clinical experience. *Journal of Nursing Education, 28,* 127–132.

Rickelman, B., Taylor-Fox, J., Reisch, J., Payne, P., & Jelemensky, L. (1988). Effect of a CVIS instructional program regarding therapeutic communication on student learning and anxiety. *Journal of Nursing Education, 27,* 312–320.

Scheetz, L. J. (1989). Baccalaureate nursing student preceptorship programs and the development of clinical competence. *Journal of Nursing Education, 28,* 29–35.

Scholdra, J. D., & Quiring, J. D. (1973). The level of questions posed by nursing educators. *Journal of Nursing Education, 12*(3), 15–20.

Schulman, J. L., Foley, J. M., & Voorsanger, E. L. (1966). Observation of a hospitalized child as a teaching technique in student nurse education. *Journal of Nursing Education, 5*(4), 7–12, 20–21.

Schwirian, P. (1978). Evaluating the performance of nurses: A multidimensional approach. *Nursing Research, 27,* 347–351.

Sedlak, C. A. (1992). Use of clinical logs by beginning nursing students and faculty to identify learning needs. *Journal of Nursing Education, 31,* 24–27.

Sieh, S., & Bell, S. (1994). Perceptions of effective clinical teachers in associate degree programs. *Journal of Nursing Education, 33,* 389–394.

Slimmer, L. W., Wendt, A., & Martinkus, D. (1990). Effect of psychiatric clinical learning site on nursing students' attitudes toward mental illness and psychiatric nursing. *Journal of Nursing Education, 29,* 127–133.

Spielberger, C., Gorsuch, R., & Lushene, R. (1970). *STAI manual for the state-trait anxiety inventory.* Palo Alto, CA: Consulting Psychologists Press.

Stein, R. F., Steele, L., Fuller, M., & Langhoff, H. F. (1972). A multi-media independent approach: For improving the teaching-learning process in nursing. *Nursing Research, 21,* 436–447.

Stuebbe, B. (1980). Student and faculty perspectives on the role of a nursing instructor. *Journal of Nursing Education, 19,* 4–9.

Sullivan, J. A., Grover, P. L., Lynaugh, J. E., & Levy, A. (1975). Video mediated self-cognition and the Amidon-Flanders Interaction Analysis Model in the training of nurse practitioners' history taking skills. *Journal of Nursing Education, 14*(3), 39–44.

Sullivan, J. A., & Weber, M. H. (1970). Nurses bag technique—self-taught. *Nursing Outlook, 18*(6), 59.

Treece, E. M. (1969). Student opinions concerning patient selection for clinical practice. *Journal of Nursing Education, 8*(2), 17–25.

Van Den Berg, E. L. (1976). The multiple student assignment: An effective alternative for laboratory experiences. *Journal of Nursing Education, 15*(3), 3–12.

Wang, A. M., & Blumberg, P. (1983). A study on interaction techniques of nursing faculty in the clinical area. *Journal of Nursing Education, 22*, 144–150.

Williams, R. P. (1993). The concerns of beginning nursing students. *Nursing & Health Care, 14*, 178–184.

Wilson, M. E. (1994). Nursing student perspective of learning in a clinical setting. *Journal of Nursing Education, 33*, 81–86.

Windsor, A. (1987). Nursing students' perceptions of clinical experience. *Journal of Nursing Education, 26*, 150–154.

Wink, D. M. (1993a). Effect of a program to increase the cognitive level of questions asked in clinical postconferences. *Journal of Nursing Education, 32*, 357–363.

Wink, D. M. (1993b). Using questioning as a teaching strategy. *Nurse Educator, 18*(5), 11–15.

Wiseman, R. F. (1994). Role model behaviors in the clinical setting. *Journal of Nursing Education, 33*, 405–410.

Wong, J., Wong, S., & Richard, J. (1994). Implementing computer simulations as a strategy for evaluating decision-making skills of nursing students. *Computers in Nursing, 10*, 264–269.

Yonge, O., & Trojan, L. (1992). The nursing performance of preceptored and non-preceptored baccalaureate nursing students. *Canadian Journal of Nursing Research, 24*(4), 61–75.

Zimmerman, L., & Westfall, J. (1988). The development and validation of a scale measuring effective clinical teaching behaviors. *Journal of Nursing Education, 27*, 274–277.

Chapter Five

SPIRITUALITY AND NURSING EDUCATION
Ruth Ann B. Fulton, DNSc, RN

Articles about spirituality began to appear in the nursing literature during the 1970s. During this period, nursing education was moving from hospital-based programs with curricula founded on the medical model toward higher education settings with curricula structured on conceptual frameworks incorporating theory across disciplines (Neuman, 1989). As the metaparadigm for nursing became known to students in nursing theory courses and as nursing conceptual frameworks guided the research process, holistic nursing practice began to free the profession from the body-mind dualism of medicine by caring for the spirit of persons.

As nursing became a discipline, refinement of nursing theory, more sophisticated research, additional scholarly journals, increased numbers of doctoral programs in nursing, and use of computers for information management strengthened the foundation for the art and science of nursing. Simultaneously, a recognition of and inquiry about the spirituality of clients, nursing students, and nurses in practice began to evolve in the literature.

The literature also reveals that nurses sometimes ignore or misinterpret spiritual needs (Ellis, 1986; Heliker, 1992; Taylor, Amenta, & Highfield, 1995), or inappropriately treat spiritual needs as psychosocial needs (Highfield & Cason, 1983; Piles, 1980, 1990). Such problems associated with lack of spiritual care may be inherent in the sensitive nature of spiritual issues, the confusion about multiple terms related to spirituality, the omission of a focus on spirituality in nursing curricula, and the lack of awareness of a personal spirituality (Buys, 1981; Carson, 1989; Dettmore, 1986; Granstrom, 1985; Hitchens, 1988). In this regard, nursing education and practice do need to recognize spirituality as a component of holistic nursing care for individuals, families, groups, and communities.

127

This chapter clarifies the concept of spirituality, explains its relevance to the education of nurses who will practice in the 21st century, discusses findings and implications of a literature review, provides a synthesis from the review, and stimulates the profession to consider research agendas about spirituality and nursing education.

CLARIFICATION OF THE CONCEPT OF SPIRITUALITY

There is no doubt that the nursing literature on spirituality lacks clarity, but this may be a reflection of the use or misuse of the concept itself. The interchangeable use of related terms of religion, spiritual dimension, spiritual well-being, spiritual care, spiritual needs, and spiritual distress add to such obscurity. Several authors have proposed that these terms are different than, but intertwined with, spirituality (Burkhardt, 1989; Stoll, 1989) and may be less confusing if they were referred to as subconcepts of spirituality (Fulton, 1995). Emblen (1992) described the nurse's role in relation to religion as "helping people maintain their belief system" and in relation to spirituality as "helping people identify meaning and purpose in their lives, maintain personal relationships, and transcend a given moment" (p. 47). Haase, Britt, Coward, Leidy, and Penn (1992) provided a simultaneous concept analysis of spiritual perspective, hope, acceptance, and self-transcendence that results in connectedness as a common theme among the four concepts. These descriptions suggest theory and research and support the need to educate nurses about the concepts "to attain a better appreciation of client experiences, enhance interprofessional communication, and encourage well-defined intervention studies critical to the development of nursing science" (p. 146).

Burkhardt (1989) presented a concept analysis of spirituality and proposed "spiriting" to be "the unfolding of mystery through harmonious interconnectedness that springs from inner strength" (p. 72). This definition captured the breadth of the concept and improved the process of assessment as the nurse is present with the client. A constructed case explains that "unfolding mystery" refers to the journey of adversity in which a person finds meaning and purpose; that "inner strength" suggests a person seeks guidance from within the self; and that "harmonious interconnectedness" includes meaningful relationships with significant others, the self, and a higher being that provides a feeling of peace (p. 74).

These and other clarifications (Fulton, 1995; Labun, 1988; Lane, 1987; Stoll, 1989) can assist educators to provide a consistency among terms used in nursing curricula, thereby reducing the problem of confusion among interrelated terms.

RELEVANCE OF SPIRITUALITY TO NURSING EDUCATIONAL PREPARATION OF NURSES FOR THE 21ST CENTURY

Optimal nursing care requires an understanding of spirituality and its subconcepts. The prediction is that in the early 21st century 51.1% of the U.S. population will be from culturally diverse origins (Swanson & Albrecht, 1993, p. 372). Leininger (1994) predicts that these cultural groups will choose to live in rural areas and other nonurban areas. Nurses should be prepared to provide care for individuals, families, groups, and communities that have varying views of health, illness, and death. Intertwined with these views are beliefs, values, and practices of a spiritual nature that are often inherent in the culture's perspective of meaning and purpose in life.

Another example of diversity in populations is evident in the increasing number of elderly persons in our society. The elderly will comprise nearly 22% of the U.S. population by 2050. This group currently is the greatest user of health and health-related services. Only 7% of this group state they have no religious affiliation (Swanson & Albrecht, 1993). These facts suggest that religion is likely to be an aspect of the spirituality of the elderly. Ebersole and Hess (1990) contend that religion provides a source of strength and coping in later life. Nurses will need to understand the spirituality of the elderly in order to provide holistic care, including spiritual needs.

Dying is a human event that includes "the spiritual component of patient care" (Spiritual Care Work Group, 1990, p. 75). A theoretical background in spiritual development and the transitional phases of the dying process is requisite to assess spiritual needs; to provide access to expressions of spirituality such as rituals, practices, and meditation; and to prevent spiritual distress (Stepnick & Perry, 1992).

In the 21st century, nurses will practice in restructured work environments, many of which are outside of hospitals and focus upon wellness and holism. Inherent in the focus on wellness and holism is spirituality (Chapman, 1986; Clark, Cross, Deane, & Lowry, 1991; Dossey, Keegan, Guzzetta, & Kolkmeier, 1995; Swinford & Webster, 1989; Vaughn, 1986).

Problems of homelessness, violence, and suicide within these populations may be amenable to interventions that include spiritual care. Donley (1991) suggested that "the reintroduction of spiritual values into the education and practice of nursing would go a long way toward restoring respect for certain categories of patients . . . the poor, persons of different races or cultures, confused, older persons, persons ill with certain diseases such as AIDS, or persons addicted to drugs or patterns of violence" and "bring greater meaning to the work of nursing" (p. 182). Similarly, Henry (1995) expressed excitement about the increased evidence that spirituality is regaining attention in institutions of higher learning, which may lead to an improvement in the moral status of our country.

REVIEW OF THE LITERATURE

Search strategies to identify literature sources included an automated CINAHL search in which the descriptors of *spiritual care, spiritual distress,* and *spirituality* were used, and a manual search for research studies and anecdotal articles. The manual search entailed seeking similar terms in tables of contents, indexes, and bibliography lists in textbooks, as well as perusing discussion sections of research studies in journals. Although this latter approach was not as successful as the CINAHL search, relevant material was acquired. An effort was made to locate fugitive literature including unpublished theses and dissertations; however, many were unobtainable.

Approximately 350 research studies, anecdotal articles, books, and book chapters were found in the search process. In addition, reports from conferences were acquired either through attendance or networking with persons in attendance. Criteria for inclusion of material for this review were a focus on (1) nursing students or faculty and spirituality, (2) nursing curricula and spirituality, or (3) implications for nursing education related to spirituality. Subsequently, the most useful kinds of material were research study reports and anecdotal articles that were supported by research findings or discussion.

Synthesis of Current Knowledge

The majority of spirituality literature centered on the concept solely or included an analysis of the subconcepts of spiritual well-being, spiritual distress, spiritual needs, and spiritual care in relation to persons experiencing selected situational life crises. For the purposes of this review, three categories of studies are presented: (1) spiritual characteristics of students and faculty, (2) inclusion of spirituality in nursing curricula, and (3) incidental findings related to spirituality and nursing education. The review is presented in chronological order to capture how the level of sophistication improved over time.

Spiritual characteristics of students and faculty.   Four studies specifically address spiritual characteristics of nursing students. Two studies included spiritual characteristics of nursing faculty.

Carson, Winkelstein, Soeken, and Brunins (1986) conducted a descriptive study to determine (1) if attitudes, values, beliefs, and practices related to spirituality of nursing students were improved as a result of an elective course about spirituality, (2) if the attitudes related to spirituality of those enrolled in the course ($n = 31$) were changed and how the change compared to students not enrolled in the course ($n = 145$), and (3) to compare the perceived religiosity of the students enrolled in the course to that of students enrolled in other health electives. The intended outcome for the elective course was "to encourage students to examine their own spirituality and be aware of the impact of religion on themselves and on the clients for whom they care . . . to appreciate the nurse's role in facilitating a client's spiritual journey" (Carson, Winkelstein, Soeken, & Brunins, 1986, p. 162).

A demographic questionnaire and the Religious Belief Questionnaire (RBQ) were administered to all students at the beginning and the end of the semester in which the course was completed. Before administration of the RBQ, students were asked to respond to questions regarding their perceptions about their religiosity. Although the authors do not specify the questions, the results suggest they were asked if they considered themselves to be religious, if their religious beliefs played a significant part in their lives, and how frequently they attended church or synagogue.

The RBQ measures attitudes, values, beliefs, and practices related to spirituality. It is comprised of 64 items that include the subscales of: (1) perceptions of God, (2) prayer, (3) the Bible, (4) good and evil and their consequences, (5) organized religion, (6) religious practices, and (7) the impact of religion on daily living. Responses to the items are scored on a five-point Likert-type scale and low scores represent "less religiosity" (Carson, Winkelstein, Soeken, & Brunins, 1986, p. 163).

No significant differences were evident among demographic variables of students in the sample. Dependent t-tests were used to compare RBQ pretest and post-test mean scores of students in the spirituality course. These findings showed an increase in subscale mean scores relating to perceptions and beliefs about God, the value of the Bible, the value of organized religion and the impact of it on one's life, and the necessity of attending religious practices. However, there was a decrease in subscale mean scores in regard to the value of prayer, the value of and consequences related to good and evil, and the impact of religious attitudes upon interacting in daily life. Analysis of covariance showed significant changes among students in the study group in the scores related to the subscales of God, the Bible, types of religions, and religious practices.

Before taking the RBQ, 64% of students stated they were religious and 76% believed their religion impacted their lives; however, only 34% attended a weekly worship service and 19% attended only monthly. Because no significant difference on the RBQ was evident between students in the spirituality elective and those who were not, the investigators concluded that the study group selected positive responses to RBQ items relevant to religion because an emphasis on religions and their impact on health care was a major part of course content. Furthermore, students' perceptions were that religion played an important role in their lives, but only one-third attend weekly worship services. This supports the idea that church attendance plays a minimal role in spirituality. Limitations in this study were the intent to measure spiritual attitudes through the use of a religious belief scale, the bias toward religion in the course content, and a convenience sample in one geographic area.

A correlational descriptive study was performed to measure graduate nursing students' ($n = 24$) and senior nursing students' ($n = 29$) attitudes about providing spiritual care (Soeken & Carson, 1986). Instruments included a demographic data questionnaire, the Spiritual Well-Being Scale (SWB), and the Health Professional's Spiritual Role Scale (HPSR). The 20-item SWB has a six-point response scale that ranges from strongly agree to strongly disagree and is comprised of the religious well-being (RWB) subscale and the existential well-being (EWB) subscale, because spiritual well-being was perceived to be a two-dimensional concept (Ellison, 1983). Ten items in the SWB pertain to a relationship with God (RWB) and the remaining 10 items pertain to psychosocial aspects (EWB) of spiritual well-being. High SWB scores denote spiritual well-being. Ellison (1983) states the SWB has demonstrated criterion validity with other variables. Frequent use of this scale has been evident in the literature and adequate reliability coefficients are stated. In the literature, this scale has been referred to as the Paloutzian and Ellison Spiritual Well-Being Scale (SWB). Other measures of spiritual well-being use differentiating acronyms.

The two-part HPSR was developed by Soeken and Carson (1986). The first part contains 28 attitudinal statements that have six possible response ranges from strongly agree to strongly disagree. For example, one item stated "Most health professionals are aware of the need to assess the spirituality of patients" (p. 53). The second part consists of 13 spiritually focused nursing behaviors to which respondents may select four responses ranging from not appropriate to very appropriate. These behaviors included praying with and for a patient, talking with and listening to a patient about religious beliefs, and showing kindness and concern toward a patient. The test was reliable in a pilot study, but no reliability data or comments about validity were provided.

Spiritual well-being of graduate and undergraduate students was positively correlated with their perceptions of the health professional's role to provide spiritual care to patients. The behaviors listed in the HPSR were considered by all students to be appropriate for health professionals. No correlation existed in either group between age and spiritual well-being, attitudes toward the spiritual role, and appropriateness of nursing behaviors related to spiritual care. No significant difference existed between number of years in practice among the graduate group of nursing students and the selected measures. Soeken and Carson (1986) concluded that nurses who have high spiritual well-being scores and who are inclined toward an interest in spiritual care of patients may be suited to become "spiritual specialists" (p. 54).

Spiritual wellness and awareness do not necessarily indicate nurses will use spiritual care interventions in their practice. The educational process should be directed toward knowing and implementing activities involved in spiritual care. Use of a convenience sample and lack of validity and reliability information about the HPSR limit the generalizability and usefulness of this study.

Deane, Cross, and Barber (1990) reported preliminary findings of a descriptive study that identified the levels of spiritual well-being and attitudes of nursing students ($n = 806$) regarding spiritual care. A demographic questionnaire, Spiritual Well-Being Scale (SWB), and the Health Professional's Spiritual Role Scale (HPSR) were used for the study. No validity and reliability statistics were stated for these instruments, although the SWB data have been published and the HPSR has been available since 1986.

Demographic data showed 25% of the sample to be associate degree students and 75% to be baccalaureate degree nursing students, 3% to be male and 97% to be female, 88% of the sample to be either Catholic or Protestant, and 54% of the sample to attend a religious service from 1 to 8 times per month. Of these variables, church attendance, age, and length of education program were correlated with spiritual well-being.

The investigators reported factor analysis results on role attitudes and behavior items that student attitudes about spiritual care and spiritual well-being were significant in a positive direction. There was a positive relationship between a high number of religious services attended and level of SWB. This finding is significant because it is not consistent with that of Carson, Winkelstein, Soeken, and Brunins (1986) who stated church attendance plays a minimal role in spirituality. Length of educational program did not influence SWB, although there was a positive relationship between age of students and SWB scores.

Deane, Cross, and Barber (1990) believe their preliminary findings suggest a need to continue clarifying the effect of teaching the role of the nurse in spiritual matters. No statements were given about the sampling method used for this study and about validity and reliability of the SWB or HPSR; therefore, results need to be interpreted with caution.

Carson, Soeken, and Grimm (1988) performed a correlational study to test the hypothesis: "There is a positive relationship between hope and spiritual well-being in a sample of healthy young adults" (p. 162). The convenience sample included junior nursing students ($n = 197$) at a university school of nursing. A demographic questionnaire, the Spiritual Well-Being Scale (SWB) and the State-Trait Hope Scale were used for the study. The SWB is subdivided into Religious Well-Being (RWB) and Existential Spiritual Well-Being (EWB). Carson, Soeken, and Grimm (1988) reported previously established test-retest reliability of the SWB to be .86 and internal consistency to be .78. They also stated that criterion validity of the SWB had been established by the developers of the scale.

The State-Trait Hope Scale was developed by Grimm in 1984. It has 40 items to which 5 responses range from strongly agree to strongly disagree. State hope is measured by 20 items on the scale that reflect the dynamic and changing dimension of hope at a given time; whereas trait hope is measured by 20 items that reflect a general feeling of hope most of the time. Test-retest reliability for the State-Trait Hope Scale during development of the instrument was reported to be .83, for state hope to be .99, and for trait hope to be .99. These results are higher than the coefficient alphas of .84 for state hope and .82 for trait hope established in the current study.

Results of the study showed a positive relationship between hope and spiritual well-being. Those persons with high hope tended to have high levels of spiritual well-being. Trait hope, which means being generally hopeful most of the time, and existential well-being, which denotes psychosocial aspects of spiritual well-being, showed a significantly stronger correlation than did trait hope and religious well-being, which refers to a relationship with God aspect of spiritual well-being. In addition, a strong correlation ($r = .862$) between state and trait hope was noted.

The authors suggested that hope is a psychological concept linked to the existential aspect of spiritual well-being. The linkage is attributed to the assumption that persons are integrated wholes of physiological, psychological, and spiritual who react to stimuli in a holistic manner. Furthermore, the authors explain that this sample of healthy young adults have hopeful attitudes that are grounded in the future expectation of becoming nurses. This age group tends to develop existential concerns, such as relationships and life satisfaction, before they are ready to become rooted in religious commitments in their lives which explains the high relationship between trait hope and existential well-being (Carson, Soeken, & Grimm, 1988). A convenience sample and lack of validity statements about the State-Trait Hope Scale limit the generalizability of the findings to this group of nursing students.

Fulton (1992) studied spiritual well-being of nursing students ($n = 225$) and nursing faculty ($n = 41$) and their perceptions about the spiritual well-being of persons. The sample was recruited from private secular, public, Protestant, and Catholic schools. Instrumentation included the JAREL Spiritual Well-Being Scale (JAREL) and a demographic data sheet which asked three open-ended questions about the spiritual well-being of persons. The JAREL is a 21-item questionnaire with responses on a 6-point Likert-type scale ranging from strongly agree to strongly disagree. During instrument development, the following three factors evolved from factor analysis of the scale: (1) Faith/Belief Dimension, or items which relate to spiritual beliefs, prayer, and belief in a higher power; (2) Life/Self-Responsibility, or items referring to forgiveness, acceptance of change in life, and decision making in life; and (3) Life Satisfaction/Self-Actualization, or items pertaining to setting goals, loving relationships, and self-esteem.

Results showed there was a significant difference between student and faculty scores ($t = 5.55$, $p < .05$) and between both groups in the Faith/Belief factor scores ($t = 6.80$, $p < .05$) and the Life/Self Responsibility scores ($t = 3.19$, $p = .05$). A regression analysis resulted in the independent variables of age and type of school as having influenced JAREL scores of nursing students, whereas no variables influenced faculty scores. Analysis of covariance showed no interaction between age and type of school, indicating they independently influenced JAREL scores. Further analysis of comparisons among types of schools showed Protestant, then Catholic, as predictors of high JAREL scores. In addition, for every increase in one year of age, there was an increase of .28 in the JAREL score. The Chronbach's alpha for this administration to 19- to 64-year-old adults was .81 compared to .85 among a group of 65- year-old and older adults (Hungelmann, Kenkel-Rossi, Klassen, & Stollenwerk, 1989). Responses to the three open-ended questions resulted in similar responses of students and faculty in describing the spiritual well-being of persons and nursing actions that affect spiritual well-being of persons. Furthermore, the responses were similar to findings in the literature. Limitations of this study include use of a newly developed instrument and the limited geographic.

Everhart (1994) performed a correlational study of spiritual well-being of nurse educators ($n = 77$) and the emphasis they place on spiritual care in teaching activities. Instrumentation included the Spiritual Well-being Scale (SWB) and the Educational Activities Assessment Tool (EAAT) that had been developed and piloted by the investigator. The EAAT included demographic data about nurse educators and eight items with responses on a 6-point scale ranging from strongly agree to strongly disagree. The items were developed from a review of the literature and focused on the nursing process as it relates to spiritual care and teaching techniques centered on spiritual care. A pilot study resulted in determining the amount of time needed to complete the questionnaire and deleting or revising several of the items. Everhart (1994) claimed the tool had face validity, but did not refer to reliability data.

Results showed "a significant positive relationship between nurse educators' scores on the SWB scale and the EAAT" (Everhart, 1994, p. 36).

Furthermore, the highest mean of the EAAT items was that nursing faculty teach use of therapeutic communication skills when teaching about spiritual care. This finding was similar to the responses of faculty regarding nursing actions that affect spiritual well-being of persons (Fulton, 1992). Convenience sampling and lack of reliability and validity of the EAAT limit the findings of Everhart's study.

Inclusion of spirituality in nursing curricula. Six studies address inclusion of spirituality into nursing curricula. Piles (1980) conducted an exploratory study to determine the extent to which spiritual care was addressed in nursing curricula in the United States. Sixty associate degree (ADN) and 60 baccalaureate degree (BSN) schools of nursing were randomly selected from the 4 major regions of the country.

A questionnaire developed by Piles (1980) was designed to assess whether schools' philosophy considered humans to be holistic and the inclusion of the spiritual dimension in this holism? A return rate of 82% showed 22 BSN schools to be state supported and 27 to be private; however, 22 of these private schools were religiously affiliated. Of the ADN schools, 45 were state-supported and 4 were religiously affiliated.

The major findings of Piles' (1980) study were: (1) the majority of ADN and BSN schools confirmed the spiritual dimension of man was in the curriculum, but it was subsumed under the psychosocial content; (2) BSN programs tended to include more questions about spiritual needs of the patient in their assessment tools than did ADN programs; (3) and the skill of use of self was reported by both types of schools to be an intervention in the presence of a spiritual need. Piles (1980) expressed concern about the tendency of nursing schools to teach nurses to treat spiritual problems with psychosocial interventions. The author considered this approach to be antithetic to nursing's claim to heal persons holistically and urged educators to realize that, although the dimensions of a person are "intertwining and interacting with each other" (p. 66), the separate and unique needs of each dimension require separate interventions. No suggestions or examples of how to intervene in each dimension were offered by Piles. The literature about spiritual care generally suggests psychosocial interventions such as touching, listening, and being compassionate. Most often, referrals to clergy, religious readings, and prayer are stated as spiritual interventions, although they are only appropriate for those who have religious beliefs. Those interventions that are mentioned that incorporate a broad perception of spirituality are the use journaling, sharing of life review, storytelling, and dream telling. These activities may reach the core, or spirit, of a person in the search for meaning and purpose in life.

The study was well-developed as evidenced by a random sample, support for the validity of the questionnaire, and a high return rate;

however, the bias of the researcher was from a Judeo-Christian perspective. The results of the study are helpful for schools that embrace Piles' (1980) belief system, and, the focus of spirituality can be adapted to fit the needs of other schools.

Dettmore (1986) conducted an exploratory study of nurses' conceptions of, and practices in the spiritual dimension of nursing and used an interview schedule of 13 questions. One of the questions asked nurses about their educational preparation in regard to the spiritual dimension and the majority stated they had "minimal to no content" (p. 141) in this area. Some subjects adapted life experiences, liberal arts learning, or role modeling experiences to their practice in order to address spiritual issues of their patients. A small number of subjects stated they "had maximal instruction in this dimension within their schools of nursing" (p. 142). These respondents claim they had theoretical, clinical, and faculty role modeling learning experiences in the spiritual dimension. The investigator concluded that the words *acting* and *reacting* best described learning situations related to the spiritual dimension. Nurses who received a strong knowledge base in the spiritual dimension were able to be active in the dimension because they could confidently provide appropriate spiritual care interventions, whereas the nurses who were less knowledgeable about the spiritual dimension reacted to the message of indifference about this dimension from their educators by providing spiritual care interventions as best they could, if at all.

Dettmore (1986) suggested two implications for nursing education: (1) spirituality is a complex concept that may need to be taught using a simple-to-complex approach, and (2) nursing faculty should be encouraged to incorporate into classroom and clinical learning the valuable experiences of philosophers, ethicists, clerics, and nurses which relate to meeting the spiritual needs of clients.

A descriptive study about the stages of faith and values development yielded implications for spiritual care involving nursing students and patients (Hitchens, 1988). A sample included 10 basic nursing students and 10 registered nurses in a baccalaureate completion track from a "protestant, evangelical" (p. 2) university. Each group was separately enrolled in a course entitled "Values, Faith Development and Spiritual Care." During the first half of the school quarter, data were compiled from demographic questionnaires, nursing care plans devised two spiritual care case studies, from individual faith development interviews, and through the use of The Personal Discernment Inventory (PDI). The remaining class sessions involved didactic and experiential teaching strategies.

The researcher analyzed data by assigning them to either emerging or integrative themes. Emerging themes were representative phrases that best captures ideas which evolved from the analysis of care plans, faith development interviews and the PDI. Integrative themes came from data which made "the connection between the giving of spiritual care and faith and value development" (Hitchens, 1988, p. 275).

Emerging themes from spiritual care case studies were that students could state a beginning level of spiritual care; students perceived developing rapport and use of self as interventions; and students believed prayer, scripture, and consulting pastoral services were important interventions. Hitchens (1988) stated that the theoretical frameworks of Fowler and Parks provided support for the major emerging theme from the faith development interviews which was: Students were experiencing faith stages that were congruent with their developmental stages. The major emerging theme from the PDI was that interpersonal values were very important to students. Integrative themes that developed from the study were that a relationship was evident between spiritual care and values and faith development; spiritual care plans reflected values, faith stages, and life experience; and interpersonal values were evident in the majority of care plans (Hitchens, 1988).

As a result of the data analysis, Hitchens (1988) developed five implications for nurse educators in reference to spiritual care. The nurse educator needs to (1) present learning experiences which assist students to adapt their faith and value development to providing spiritual care; (2) emphasize the development and use of therapeutic communication skills as they pertain to spiritual care; (3) provide essential background information about the nursing process with an emphasis on diagnosing spiritual distress and developing spiritual care interventions; (4) provide the use of experiential, reflecting activities which promote an awareness of a personal spiritual journey; and (5) and enhance the use of interpersonal skills as an important intervention in spiritual care. A small convenience sample and the use of tools that are highly subjective in nature limited the study. Findings cannot be generalized beyond this study group.

Schnorr (1988) performed an exploratory pilot study to determine how many schools of nursing in Illinois ($n = 45$) had the concept of spirituality in their curricula and to determine how many schools taught content about spiritual care. Of the 50% of the questionnaires that were returned, all stated they at least mentioned spirituality in the curriculum; however, only 40% stated they taught about spiritual care. Subsequently, the investigator developed 59 specific objectives about spiritual care which could be integrated into the theoretical and practical aspects of nursing courses. Similarly, a detailed plan for course content of an elective in spirituality was developed. These materials were planned for use in the investigator's next step of research which is to offer, distribute, implement, and evaluate the use of the plans to teach spiritual care in schools of nursing in Illinois.

In an exploratory study by Piles (1990), practicing nurses were asked to identify the amount of time spent on spirituality related content in their educational preparation. Nurses were also asked about their perceived ability to adequately meet spiritual needs of patients, their opinions about the nurse's role in this area, and their perceptions about obstacles which prevented them from providing spiritual care. A stratified random sample of practicing registered nurses was obtained from the four regions of the United States. A 5-point Likert scale questionnaire with questions pertaining to spiritual needs, spiritual care, and educational content on spirituality was sent to 300 nurses. A 59% return rate with relatively equal distribution among the four regions was obtained.

Findings were significant at a $p < .001$ level with use of the Kendall Tau C and Pearson Correlation Coefficient statistical tests. Specifically, the findings showed significant relationships between level of practice (of spiritual care) and perceived ability to provide care, level of practice and amount of educational preparation time in this area, and level of practice and obstacles (lack of time and lack of knowledge) in preventing provision of spiritual care. A multiple regression analysis was used to determine the prediction of the variables of ability, education, opinion, and obstacles on the extent of spiritual care provided by practicing nurses. Ability, education, and opinion accounted for nearly two-thirds of the variance in perceived practice and, therefore, may be the strongest predictors. Ninety-seven percent of the nurses believed spiritual care to be an aspect of holistic care, 88% disagreed that only clergy were capable of providing spiritual care, and 66% believed they were inadequately prepared to assess and act appropriately to an expressed spiritual need. Differences between spiritual and psychosocial needs were not delineated in 58% of the respondents' education programs, and differences in specific interventions in these areas were not addressed in 66% of the respondents' educational programs. Lack of time and lack of knowledge were perceived as the two greatest obstacles to providing spiritual care. The inclusion of spiritual care content in every nursing curriculum was agreed upon by 89% of the nurses who responded to the survey.

Piles' (1990) findings are similar to those of other studies in the nursing literature which suggest spiritual needs of the patients may be identified as psychosocial needs and, therefore, spiritual needs are not met (Carson, Winkelstein, Soeken, & Brunins 1986; Highfield & Cason, 1983; Piles, 1980, 1990; Soeken & Carson, 1986). This study is important because of the use of a random sample and because the findings support previous studies.

In a descriptive study, Fulton (1992) found baccalaureate nursing students stated coursework pertaining to the spiritual well-being of persons was either integrated into their coursework, or addressed in clinical experiences, or incorporated into theory about holistic persons. Faculty stated similar responses. Although no information was given related to the quantity and quality of these learning experiences, the findings suggest spiritual well-being of persons is addressed to some degree in nursing curricula.

Incidental findings related to spirituality and nursing education. Studies about spirituality in the nursing literature that did not necessarily focus on the relevance of spirituality and nursing education either noted incidental findings related to nursing education or concluded that the findings had implications for nursing education. Several examples are: (a) Highfield and Cason (1983) implied that nursing education curricula should distinguish between spiritual problems and psychosocial problems of patients because practicing nurses in their study did not perceive a difference between these two concepts; (b) Boutell and Bozett (1990) suggest that continuing education about spirituality is needed to provide nurses with an ability to recognize spiritual aspects of nursing care; and (c) Hall and Lanig (1993) believe their study suggests research is needed to determine factors that facilitate preparing nurses to give spiritual care.

There is evidence in other health professions that spirituality is not being addressed in educational programs and in practice. For example, the social work literature addresses lack of education about spirituality in social work education (Canda, 1988; Joseph, 1988). In the health education literature, the concept of spirituality is in a beginning phase of development.

Banks (1980) used an adaptation of the Delphi technique to determine how health educators perceived the spiritual dimension of health and the extent to which it should be incorporated into curricula. This approach involved three rounds of data collection. The investigator found the majority of health educators supported a belief in the existence of the spiritual dimension of persons and wanted to include the dimension in program curricula. The highest ranked components of the spiritual dimension were meaning or purpose to life, a set of principles to abide by, and a sense of selflessness. The highest ranked ideas to be considered when teaching about the dimension were to recognize a diversity of backgrounds in groups of students, have respect for other persons' opinions about the dimension, and acknowledge a variety of spiritual belief systems. Uses of problem solving, valuing, and judgment situations were the highest rankings of teaching methodologies. Second and third rankings were use of a holistic approach and group work.

Another article synthesized research (Banks, Poehler, & Russell, 1984) to develop a list of findings about spirituality and health education. The assertions can be summarized as follows: First, the spirit of a person is a reality reflecting a state of well-being through human-spirit interactions that contribute to positive health. Second, the spiritual dimension should be part of health education curricula with particular sensitivity to the diversity of differences persons value in terms of importance. Third, religious beliefs and practices may or may not be incorporated into a person's spiritual dimension. Fourth, meaning and purpose in life are closely aligned to the spirit of the person. Fifth, caring, sharing and acting in a selfless manner are descriptive terms that identify the spiritual dimension of a person. Sixth, concern outside of self may be linked to others, groups, God in the abstract form, or God through a relationship with Jesus Christ and/or the Holy Spirit. Seventh, the spirit is considered as the unifier of relationships and of the holistic self. Eighth, a manifestation of the spirit is often described as an inner strength. Ninth, an acknowledgment may be made about communicating with God, other "disembodied spirits" (p. 19), and nature. Tenth, a recognition by respondents may be described as having a personal relationship with Jesus Christ through faith. This last assertion has been described as the most controversial.

Banks, Poehler, and Russell (1984) conclude that their work developed a foundation in the health education research literature about spirituality. Also, there exists a need to continue research about the spiritual dimension of persons and to explore human-spiritual interaction in the context of the health education profession. Banks (1980) and Banks, Poehler, and Russell (1984) are frequently cited in nursing literature for the relevance of their work to nursing education. These findings are congruent with the theoretical work of Stoll (1989) and Neuman (1995), and the studies of Hungelmann, Kenkel-Rossi, Klassen, and Stollenwerk (1985; 1989), as well as Dossey, Keegan, Guzzetta, and Kolkmeier (1995) and the holistic nursing literature.

STATE OF THE SCIENCE

Research on spirituality and nursing education has emerged in the literature during the 1980s and 1990s. Very few studies have been published, although the "fugitive" literature suggests a larger number of studies are in the form of theses and dissertations. The "fugitive" literature was determined through the author's perusal of thesis and dissertation titles published by the Nurses Christian Fellowship and dissertation titles published by Sigma Theta Tau International Honor Society of Nursing and their comparison to the published research titles. This section is intended to stimulate nurse educators to consider the relevance of spirituality to nursing practice and to motivate researchers to develop agendas that will add to the limited existing knowledge base.

This comprehensive review of literature about spirituality points to the implications for nursing curricula, teaching strategies, and nursing practice. The implications are difficult to separate and relegate to any single title, therefore the conclusions are presented as a whole. This difficulty is related to the numerous descriptors in the literature given for the concept of spirituality.

Health education and nursing literature suggests students perceive a need for and desire knowledge about the spiritual dimension of their clients. The anecdotal nursing literature provides implications for nursing research about spirituality, especially the references to the spiritual needs of persons, the characteristics of spiritual distress, and the nursing interventions related to spiritual care. Until these ideas of authors are supported by research, it is difficult to include them in nursing education content that relates to spirituality

Empirical studies about spirituality and its relevance to education of health professionals show development of a knowledge base in this area. New and researchable questions arise from this emerging knowledge. The most common finding from nursing studies is that, in the event a nursing program includes spirituality and related subconcepts in the curriculum, the concepts are often subsumed under psychosocial content. The result may likely be that patients who have spiritual needs may not have those needs met by nurses using psychosocial interventions. It follows that psychosocial interventions may be frequently used instead of interventions which promote spiritual well-being in crises and during wellness. Another common finding suggests nursing students who possess spiritual well-being are optimistic about the future and perceive themselves as capable of providing spiritual care to their patients.

A synthesis of the findings from the majority of spirituality studies suggests that persons who profess to have a sense of their own spirituality may be better equipped to deal with difficult life situations than those who have a minimal or no sense of their own spirituality. This is a tenuous statement because participants in studies related to spirituality tend to be members of religions with a Judeo-Christian heritage. Research is needed to determine the spirituality of persons who have no religious affiliation and express their spiritual dimension through a humanistic philosophy. For these persons, the research question might be "Is it appropriate to incorporate spiritual needs into psychosocial needs?" For example, Burnard (1988a, 1988b) believes nurses are confused about the association of spiritual concerns with anything other than religion. Burnard (1988c) presents the spiritual needs of agnostics and atheists and suggests a search for meaning in life to be a nonreligious focus of spirituality.

Methodological problems in the majority of studies are the result of convenience sampling and limited geographic areas which create homogeneous, rather than heterogeneous groups. Generalizations about spirituality research need to be considered with caution. Many studies center on the Judeo-Christian religions and results are strongly biased in religiosity, rather than spirituality. A few studies do not report reliability and validity information about instruments used in research projects. This last problem is supported by Ellerhorst-Ryan (1985) and Soeken (1989) who encourage researchers in spirituality to develop reliable and valid instruments which address the multidimensionality of spirituality.

An adequate number of strategies are evident in the nursing literature for practicing nurses and nursing students to begin to examine and develop their own spirituality so they are prepared to offer spiritual care to patients. The majority of these authors suggest experiential learning techniques to develop an awareness of the participant's quest for meaning in life (Burnard, 1988a; Buys, 1981; Dossey, Keegan, Guzzetta, & Kolkmeier, 1995; Hitchens, 1988; Shelly & Fish, 1988), thoughts and feelings about illness and suffering (Boutell & Bozett, 1990; Clifford & Gruca, 1987; Ellis, 1986; Forshee, Wiebe, Siegel, Ayers, & Bacon, 1984; Nagai-Jacobson & Burkhardt, 1989; Shelly & Fish, 1988), sexuality and drug abuse (Richardson & Nolan, 1984), and a personal perception of dying (Jacik, 1989; Shelly & Fish, 1988; Taylor & Ferszt, 1990). Some of the authors avoid the use of religious language in these strategies because they believe a religious orientation is not a necessary component to teach about the spiritual dimension. A suggestion common in this literature is to use an inventory of spiritual beliefs to help the nurse be attuned to and respectful of the spiritual lives of patients. A second recurring suggestion is for educators to assess their own spirituality and have a sense of comfort with the use of experiential strategies in the classroom situation.

RECOMMENDATIONS FOR FUTURE RESEARCH

The nursing and health professions' literature provides a number of textbooks that incorporate spirituality, nursing diagnoses related to spirituality, and nursing process that stimulate critical thinking about the topic. In addition, instrumentation is available to operationalize subconcepts of spirituality (Fulton, 1995) and new instruments are being created.

A focus in nursing education research is needed to continue the growth of a knowledge base. This approach has the potential to meet the spiritual needs of diverse populations, equip graduating nurses for the 21st century, and explore new roles for nurses in a rapidly changing health care system. Recommendations are: (a) develop instruments to operationalize the spirituality subconcepts of spiritual needs, spiritual well-being, spiritual distress, and spiritual care; (b) determine and develop spiritual self-awareness of students and faculty before attempting to understand and meet spiritual needs of others; (c) determine effectiveness of strategies that promote spiritual awareness of students and faculty; (d) describe components of spiritual care across nursing curricula and appropriate teaching methods for achieving these components; (e) determine effectiveness of nursing interventions related to spiritual care provided by nursing students; (f) distinguish between spiritual care interventions and psychosocial care interventions; and (g) reduce the religious bias in research on spirituality.

REFERENCES

Banks, R. L. (1980). Health and the spiritual dimension: Relationships and implications for professional preparation programs. *Journal of School Health, 50,* 195–202.

Banks, R. L., Poehler, D. L., & Russell, R. D. (1984). Spirit and human-spirit interactions as a factor in health and in health education. *Health Education, 50*(5), 16–19.

Boutell, K. A., & Bozett, F. W. (1990). Nurses' assessment of patients' spirituality: Continuing education implications. *Journal of Continuing Education in Nursing, 21*(4), 172–176.

Burkhardt, M. A. (1989). Spirituality: An analysis of the concept. *Holistic Nursing Practice, 3*(3), 69–77.

Burnard, P. (1988a). Searching for meaning. *Nursing Times, 84*(37), 34, 36.

Burnard, P. (1988b). Discussing spiritual issues with clients. *Health Visitor, 61,* 371–372.

Burnard, P. (1988c). The spiritual needs of atheists and agnostics. *The Professional Nurse, 4*(3), 130, 132.

Buys, A. M. (1981). Discussion series sensitizes nurses to patients' spiritual needs. *Hospital Progress, 62*(10), 44, 45.

Canda, E. B. (1988). Spirituality, religious diversity, and social work practice. *Social Casework: Journal of Contemporary Social Work, 69,* 238–247.

Carson, V. B. (1989). Spirituality and the nursing process. In V. B. Carson (Ed.), *Spiritual dimensions in nursing practice* (pp. 150–179). Philadelphia: Lippincott.

Carson, V. B., Soeken, K. L., & Grimm, P. M. (1988). Hope and its relationship to spiritual well-being. *Journal of Psychology and Theology, 16*(2), 159–167.

Carson, V. B., Winkelstein, M., Soeken, K., & Brunins, M. (1986). The effect of didactic teaching in spiritual attitudes. *Image, 18,* 161–164.

Chapman, L. S. (1986). Spiritual health: A component missing from health promotion. *Journal of Health Promotion, 1*(1), 38–41.

Clark, C. C., Cross, J. R., Deane, D. M., & Lowry, L. W. (1991). Spirituality: Integral to quality care. *Journal of Holistic Practice, 5*(3), 67–76.

Clifford, M., & Gruca, J. A. (1987). Facilitating spiritual care in the rehabilitation setting. *Rehabilitation Nursing, 12,* 331–333.

Deane, D., Cross, J. R., & Barber, S. (November, 1990). *Spiritual well-being and role attitudes of nurses.* Paper presented at Third Biennial Neuman Systems Model International Symposium, Dayton, OH.

Dettmore, D. (1986). *Nurses' conceptions of and practices in the spiritual dimension of nursing.* Unpublished doctoral dissertation, Columbia University Teachers' College, New York, NY.

Donley, R. (1991). Spiritual dimensions in health care. *Nursing and Health Care, 12*(4), 178–183.

Dossey, B. M., Keegan, L., Guzzetta, C. E., & Kolkmeier, L. G. (1995). *Holistic nursing: A handbook for practice* (2nd ed.). Rockville, MD: Aspen.

Ebersole, P., & Hess, P. (1990). *Toward healthy aging: Human needs and human responses.* St. Louis: Mosby.

Ellerhorst-Ryan, J. (1985). Selecting an instrument to measure spiritual distress. *Oncology Nursing Forum, 12,* 93–94, 99.

Ellis, C. (1986). Course prepares nurses to meet patients' spiritual needs. *Hospital Progress, 67,* 76–77.

Ellison, C. W. (1983). Spiritual well-being: Conceptualization and measurement. *Journal of Psychology and Theology, 11*(4), 330–440.

Emblen, J. D. (1992). Religion and spirituality defined according to current use in nursing literature. *Journal of Professional Nursing, 8*(1), 41–47.

Everhart, N. (1994). *The relationship between a nurse educator's spiritual well-being and the emphasis he/she places on spiritual care in teaching activities.* Unpublished master's thesis. Edinboro University, Edinboro, PA.

Forshee, T., Wiebe, S., Siegel, M. A., Ayers, A. B., & Bacon, J. M. (1984). How to teach spiritual care. *Journal of Christian Nursing, 1,* 20–23.

Fulton, R. A. (1992). *Spiritual well-being of baccalaureate nursing students and faculty and their responses about well-being of persons.* Unpublished doctoral dissertation. Widener University, Chester, PA.

Fulton, R. A. (1995). The spiritual variable: Essential to the client system. In B. Neuman (Ed.), *The Neuman Systems Model* (3rd ed.). Norwalk, CT: Appleton & Lange.

Granstrom, S. L. (1985). Spiritual nursing care for oncology patients. *Topics in Clinical Nursing, 7*(1), 39–45.

Haase, J. E., Britt, T., Coward, D. D., Leidy, N. K., & Penn, P. (1992). Simultaneous concept analysis of spiritual perspective, hope, acceptance and self-transcendence. *Image, 24*(2), 141–147.

Hall, C., & Lanig, H. (1993). Spiritual caring behaviors as reported by Christian nurses. *Western Journal of Nursing Research. 15*(6), 730–741.

Heliker, D. (1992). Reevaluation of a nursing diagnosis: Spiritual distress. *Nursing Forum, 27*(4), 15–20.

Henry, B. (1995). The spiritual in nursing. *Image, 27*(3), 86.

Highfield, M. F., & Cason, C. (1983). Spiritual needs of patients: Are they recognized? *Cancer Nursing, 6,* 187–192.

Hitchens, E. W. (1988). *Stages of faith and values development and their implications for dealing with spiritual care in the student nurse-patient relationship.* Unpublished doctoral dissertation, Seattle University, Seattle, WA.

Hungelmann, J., Kenkel-Rossi, E., Klassen, L., & Stollenwerk, R. (1985). Spiritual well-being in older adults: Harmonious interconnectedness. *Journal of Religion and Health, 24,* 147–153.

Hunglemann, J., Kenkel-Rossi, E., Klassen, L., & Stollenwerk, R. (1989). Development of the JAREL Spiritual Well-Being Scale. In R. M. Carroll-Johnson (Ed.), *Classification of nursing diagnoses: Proceedings of the eighth conference* (pp. 393–398). Philadelphia: Lippincott.

Jacik, M. (1989). Spiritual care of the dying adult. In V. B. Carson (Ed.), *Spiritual dimensions of nursing practice* (pp. 254–288.). Philadelphia: Saunders.

Joseph, M. V. (1988). Religion and social work practice. *Social Casework: The Journal of Contemporary Social Work, 69,* 443–452.

Labun, E. (1988). Spiritual care: An element in nursing. *Journal of Advanced Nursing, 13,* 314–320.

Lane, J. A. (1987). The care of the human spirit. *Journal of Professional Nursing, 3,* 332–337.

Leininger, M. (November, 1994). *Coherence of culture: Caring and cost.* Keynote address at the Robert Packer Hospital First Annual Nursing Research Conference, Sayre, PA.

Nagai-Jacobson, M. G., & Burkhardt, M. A. (1989). Spirituality: Cornerstone of holistic nursing practice. *Journal of Holistic Nursing Practice, 3*(3), 18–26.

Neuman, B. (1989). *The Neuman Systems Model* (2nd ed.). Norwalk, CT: Appleton & Lange.

Neuman, B. (1995). *The Neuman Systems Model* (3rd ed.). Norwalk, CT: Appleton & Lange.

Piles, C. L. (1980). *Spiritual care as a part of the nursing curriculum: A descriptive study.* Unpublished master's thesis, St. Louis University, St. Louis, MO.

Piles, C. L. (1990). Providing spiritual care. *Nurse Educator, 15*(1), 36–41.

Richardson, G. E., & Nolan, M. P. (1984). Treating the spiritual dimension through imagery. *Health Values, 8*(6) 25–30.

Schnorr, M. A. (1988). *Spiritual nursing care: Theory and curriculum development.* Unpublished doctoral dissertation, Northern Illinois University, DeKalb, IL.

Shelly, J. A., & Fish, S. (1988). *Spiritual care: The nurse's role* (3rd ed.). Downers Grove, IL: InterVarsity.

Soeken, K. L. (1989). Perspectives on research in the spiritual dimension of nursing care. In V. B. Carson (Ed.), *Spiritual dimensions of nursing practice* (pp. 354–378). Philadelphia: Saunders.

Soeken, K. L., & Carson, V. J. (1986). Study measures nurses' attitudes about providing spiritual care. *Health Progress, 67*(3), 52–55.

Spiritual Care Work Group (1990). Assumptions and principles of spiritual care. *Death Studies, 14,* 75–81.

Stepnick, A., & Perry, T. (1992). Preventing spiritual distress in the dying client. *Journal of Psychosocial Nursing, 30*(1), 17–20.

Stoll, R. I. (1989). The essence of Spirituality. In V. B. Carson (Ed.), *Spiritual dimensions of nursing practice* (pp. 4–23). Philadelphia: Saunders.

Swanson, J. M., & Albrecht, M. (1993). *Community health nursing: Promoting the health of aggregates.* Philadelphia: Saunders.

Swinford, P. A., & Webster, J. A. (1989). *Promoting wellness.* Rockville, MD: Aspen.

Taylor, E. J., Amenta, M., & Highfield, M. (1995). Spiritual care practices of oncology nurses. *Oncology Nursing Forum, 22*(1), 31–39.

Taylor, P. B., & Ferszt, G. G. (1990). Spiritual healing. *Holistic Nursing Practice, 4*(4), 32–38.

Vaughn, F. (1986). *The inward arc: Healing and wholeness in psychotherapy and spirituality.* Boston: Shambahala.

Chapter Six

UTILIZATION OF MASTER'S AND DOCTORAL PROGRAM GRADUATES: IMPLICATIONS FOR CURRICULA

Betsy Frank, PhD, RN

The American health care system is in a dramatic period of change. More health care is being delivered in interdisciplinary managed care settings. Furthermore, the percentage of elderly seeking health care will continue to increase.

Through its *Agenda for Health Care Reform* (American Nurses Association, 1992), nursing has identified that all nurses, especially those with post-baccalaureate degrees, should and can have a central role in the restructured system.

The history of master's and doctoral education has been well-documented elsewhere (Brown, 1978; Hudacek & Carpenter, 1994). However, a need exists for assessing current utilization of and future needs for nurses with graduate degrees to help educators plan for curricula that meet the demands of the turbulent health care environment.

In order to evaluate utilization and demand for nurses with advanced degrees, both Medline and CINAHL searches were conducted via on-line and CD-ROM searches. The years 1978–1992 were searched in Medline using the descriptors "masters and doctoral programs." These same descriptors were used for the 1983–1994 CINAHL search. Older articles were located through bibliographic references cited in retrieved information. Additionally, a CINAHL search was conducted using the descriptors "graduate nursing education/evaluation." This limited search yielded 24 references, not all of which were pertinent. Finally, since nurse practitioners and clinical nurse specialists will play integral roles in a reformed health care system, a CD-ROM Medline search using the years 1990–1994 was conducted using the "nurse practitioner" and "clinical nurse specialist" role descriptor terms.

One problem encountered during the literature search was that national data sets that described the utilization of advanced practice nurses, including those with graduate degrees, were often contained in government documents not printed by the Government Printing Office.

148

Thus, their existence may have been known only to private sources or may have been referenced in published articles, but not easily located through traditional catalogues of government documents. For example, the Indiana State Nurses Association was contacted for information regarding the existence of national data sets concerned with employment characteristics of Registered Nurses with graduate degrees. The most current documents from the Health Resources and Services Administration (1994a; 1994b) were located through this source. Because the documents were so current, they were not as yet in the catalogues of government documents.

Guided by national data sets, articles were placed into the categories of current employment patterns, general role preparation, and specific role preparation. Tables 6.1 thru 6.6 summarize the literature reviewed.

CURRENT EMPLOYMENT PATTERNS

According to *The Registered Nurse Population: Findings from the National Sample of Registered Nurses, March 1992* (Health Resources and Services Administration, 1994a), an estimated 175,888 or 7.5% of registered nurses have their master's degree in nursing or a related field. Master's prepared nurses function as educators, administrators, and advanced practice clinicians (see Table 6.1).

The Health Resources and Services Administration (1994a) also estimated that 11,300 nurses have doctoral degrees and, as with those with master's degrees, not all of those are in nursing (see Table 6.2). Only 7% are involved in clinical practice as their major employment focus and over 70% are employed in education or research positions. The majority of doctorally prepared educators work in baccalaureate and

Table 6.1 Numbers of Master's and Doctorally Prepared Nurses

Practice Focus	Master's Degree Number	Doctoral Degree Number
Total	175,888[1]	11,300[1]
Clinical Practice	76,281[1,2]	774[1]
Education	11,533[3]	3,867[3]
Research	163[1]	3,721[1]
Administration	42,245[1]	946[1]

[1] Health Resources and Services Administration (1994a)
[2] Includes all advanced nurse practitioners
[3] Rosenfeld (1993)

Table 6.2   Current Employment Patterns

Author/Date	Sample	Method	Findings
Brimmer, 1983	1,964 RNs with doctorates	Investigator designed survey	Most employed in baccalaureate and higher degree programs
Health Resources & Services Administration, 1994a	National sample survey	Differential state sampling— investigator designed	Reports 50 state employment patterns as national aggregate data
Rosenfeld, 1993	National sample of all nursing faculty	Investigator designed	Reports employment patterns and demographic characteristics of nursing faculty

higher degree programs (Rosenfeld, 1993). These figures haven't changed much from research conducted in the early 1980s. At that time, a survey of the entire population of doctorally prepared nurses revealed that 76% of the 1,964 respondents worked in academic institutions (Brimmer et al., 1983).

GENERAL ROLE PREPARATION

What is expected of those who have completed graduate programs in nursing helps faculty to plan and implement appropriate curricula. The only studies found concerning general role preparation dealt exclusively with master's graduates (see Table 6.3). Studies outlining expectations of doctoral program graduates concerned preparation for the educator and researcher roles only.

An early study delineated essential competencies for master's prepared nurses (McLane, 1978). From a thorough literature review, a reliable and valid questionnaire was developed. A large random sample of deans, directors of graduate programs, and selected students from each program lent much credibility to the study's findings; but, the number of respondents in each subgroup was not identified. All respondents designated 25 items on the questionnaire as core competencies. McLane classified the core competencies into interpersonal, research, accountability, change agent, educator, and humanizer categories. While this study was reported almost 20 years ago, many of the expected competencies remain today.

Hill (1989) conducted a needs assessment for the purpose of planning a new master's program. Although not explicitly stated, Hill

Table 6.3 General Role Preparation

Author/Date	Sample	Method	Findings
Burns et al., 1993	175 Master's programs	Descriptive, investigator designed instrument	Curricula designed around multiple specialties and functional areas
Heller, Damrosch, Romano, & McCarthy, 1989	128 Nursing directors 188 Generic BSN 74 RN BSN 315 Staff nurses 30 Journal readers	Descriptive, investigator designed survey	Strong interest expressed for informatics skills
Hill, 1989	13 Administrators 34 Staff nurses	Descriptive, investigator designed survey	Interdisciplinary program recommended
Hungler, Joyce, Krawczyk, & Polit, 1979	272 Master's graduates	Theoretically based investigator designed survey	Educators scored higher on measures of professionalism
McLane, 1978	133 Deans, directors of nursing, & graduate students	Investigator designed survey	25 core competencies identified
Smith, M., 1980	37 Graduates 20 employers	Investigator designed program evaluation	Useful coursework and skills described areas for improvement identified

implied all registered nurses within a 60-mile radius of the university who held a baccalaureate degree or higher were surveyed, resulting in a responding sample size of 47. Statements from a previous Delphi survey were used to construct a questionnaire containing 18 predictive statements concerning the health care system in the year 2000. Participants estimated the probability of occurrence for each statement and suggested program content areas. Based on survey results and the higher education climate in the state, the author recommended starting an interdisciplinary masters' program with content in leadership, communication, counseling, and nursing theory. As recommended by study participants, master's level gerontology content was not included. Considering the changing demographics in the United States, this advice is somewhat perplexing. However, working within interdisciplinary environments will be a requirement of all nurses with graduate degrees. Therefore, all nursing faculty might consider ways to provide interdisciplinary experiences for students, while at the same time incorporating opportunities for exploration of the richness of advanced nursing knowledge.

One particular skill, not identified by McLane or Hill, was competency with informatics. Heller, Damrosch, Romano, and McCarthy (1989) assessed the need for a master's program with an emphasis on informatics as applied to the field of nursing. A regional sample of nurse executives, students, and staff nurses from selected academic/research hospitals, and readers of 1987 issues of *Computers in Nursing* ($n = 735$) were surveyed regarding their perceived need and interest in a master's program with an informatics specialty. Survey results and letters of endorsement lead to curriculum planning. While this survey was primarily regional, faculty might use these results as well as other clinical realities to incorporate informatics technology into every graduate program.

Specific needs assessments, whether on a national or local level, are useful in curriculum planning. Knowing what already exists in master's education on a nationwide basis can give faculty more information on which to support decisions regarding curricula. Burns et al. (1993) provided a useful database for faculty. These researchers sought to determine program admission requirements and curricular organization through an examination of written documents sent to prospective students. More than 99% of the 176 master's programs responded to the mail survey. Results indicated that required semester credit hours ranged from 29 to 59 with a mean of 36 hours of credit. Eighty-eight percent required a BSN for admission and most required a 3.0 GPA and at least one year of clinical practice. Only 4% required computer literacy for admission. More than 50% also required some pre-admission standardized test such as the Graduate Records Exam (GRE). Burns et al. concluded that multiple models existed for master's education and no consensus was present for functional role preparation for administrators or educators. They also noted that the nature of the expected research competency for master's graduates was less than clear from the written materials. Identified gaps in curricula included lack of course work on health policy. An additional recommendation was that the American Association of Colleges of Nursing (AACN) should develop a document regarding essential content and skills for master's education. Such a document, similar in scope to the AACN document concerning essentials of baccalaureate education, could complement current accreditation guidelines and might help faculty to elucidate core content required for advanced nursing practice.

Surveys of graduates and employers are a common way to evaluate the use and effectiveness of graduates. However, only two rather old studies were found which reported graduates' and employers' evaluation of master's graduates' general role performance (Hungler, Krawczyk, Joyce, & Polit, 1979; Smith, 1980). Hungler et al. (1979) surveyed graduates from one school using a questionnaire grounded in Flexner's criteria for professionalism. They discovered those in the educator role displayed more professional behaviors than did clinicians. Hungler et al. speculated that more incentives for professional behaviors existed for educators and encouraged faculty to investigate ways curricula could include strategies to stimulate an increase in professional behaviors for all graduates. Their advice seems quite timely more than 15 years later.

Smith's (1980) findings seemed to corroborate those of Hungler et al. (1979). She found that employers rated graduates' leadership behaviors somewhat lower than did the graduates themselves. One particular strength of this study was its inclusion of the survey instrument which could be used in other follow-up studies of master's graduates.

NURSE PRACTITIONERS AND
CLINICAL NURSE SPECIALISTS

The focus of the aforementioned studies was general. Utilization and effectiveness issues may also be analyzed by examining specific roles within which graduates function. The purpose of this exploration would be an identification of strengths, weaknesses, and gaps in current curricular models. Table 6.4 summarizes literature regarding specific role preparation for advanced clinical practice roles.

A recent national survey estimated 37,963 nurses were certified as nurse practitioners (NPs) or clinical nurse specialists (CNSs) (Health Resources and Services Administration, 1994b). Only 40% of NPs were master's prepared, while almost 100% of CNSs were prepared as such. One might expect the number of NPs with master's degrees to rise as certification requirements change to require master's preparation. The majority of the certified nurses (33%) was prepared exclusively as family nurse practitioners and more than 7,300 were educated exclusively as clinical specialists. Survey participants identified a multiplicity of specific practice settings and clinical foci.

Primary care is one cornerstone of health care reform. Nurse practitioners have a vital role to play in the provision of primary health care services. Knowing how practitioners are used will help nurse educators to plan appropriate educational programs. Cruikshank and Lakin (1986) found that nonmaster's prepared pediatric nurse practitioners (PNPs) were more likely to be employed in nonhospital settings, and over 50% of the master's prepared graduates had faculty roles. Since master's graduates were more mobile, the authors concluded that these graduates had a greater variety of job opportunities. The authors made no attempt to compare effectiveness of performance, but stated that the actual patient care activities did not differ between master's

Table 6.4 Nurse Practitioners, Clinical Nurse Specialists, and Other Advanced Nurse Practitioners

Author/Date	Sample	Method	Findings
Baradell, 1994	Not Applicable	Literature review	Demonstrated cost effectiveness of CNSs
Barkauskas & Blaha, 1989	98 master's programs	Investigator designed survey	32 programs considering home care majors or courses
Brophy, Rankin, Butler, & Egenes, 1989	23 hospitals	Investigator designed interview and written survey	CNSs have administrative duties and need broad range of theory and skills
Christensen, Richard, Froberg, McGovern, & Abanobi, 1985	73 MS prepared occupational health nurses	Investigator designed survey	OHNs participate in organizational decision making
Cruikshank & Lakin, 1986	112 graduates of combined certificate/MS NP program	Investigator designed survey based on prior surveys	Certificate graduates employed in primary care; MS prepared serve as faculty
Derstine, 1992	18 rehabilitation CNS graduates 5 employers	Telephone and mail investigator designed survey	Only 3 graduates functioned as CNSs; Others used knowledge in broader context Employers said graduates met program objectives
Dunn, 1993 (a, b)	Random sample of 800 NAPNAP members (520 responded)	Investigator designed survey	38.5% have MS degree Members are meeting primary health care needs of children in underserved areas
Elder & Bullough, 1990	28 CNS graduates 46 NP graduates	Investigator designed survey based on literature and practice patterns	Both groups function in similar ways
Fenton, 1992	34 MS RNs	Ethnographic	8 work role competencies explained
Fenton & Brykczynski, 1993	242 CNS clinical situations 199 NP clinical situations	Secondary analysis of qualitative data	NP's have one added domain of practice. Other domains similar
Forbes, Rafson, Spross, & Koslowski, 1990	108 master's programs	Investigator designed survey	NP and CNS programs more alike than different

Table 6.4 *(Continued)*

Author/Date	Sample	Method	Findings
Gallagher, Spross, & Powell, 1992	153 oncology CNSs 144 oncology CNSs	Two round Delphi	Clinical focus an important part of practice
Guzik, McGovern, & Kochevar, 1992	65 occupational health nurses	Investigator designed survey; descriptive correlational	Internal consultants provide more direct care. External consultants have more administrative tasks
Health Resources and Services Administration, 1990	National data bases	Projection of supply and demand	Outlined projected needs for advanced nurse practitioners
Louis & Sabo, 1994	68 nurse administrators 42 NPs 323 MDs	Investigator designed survey based on State Board of Nursing protocols	49.7% willing to hire NPs. NP group most likely to hire and MD group least likely
Mahoney, 1994	373 MDs 296 NPs	Clinical judgment of case vignettes	NPs displayed more appropriate practice decisions
McGovern, Richard, Christensen, Froberg, & Abanobi, 1985	73 occupational health nurses	Investigator designed survey	77% employed in occupational health settings. Engaged in management, teaching, and direct care roles
Radke, McArt, Schmitt, & Walker, 1990	46 CNS graduates	Investigator designed survey	CNSs participate in a variety of administrative tasks
Ramsey, Edwards, Lenz, Odom, & Brown, 1993	101 patients	Investigator designed survey	Patients very satisfied with care
Segall & McKay, 1984	43 community health graduates	Investigator designed survey	Aggregate based learning very useful. Graduates wanted more administrative content
Selby, Riportella-Muller, Salmon, Legault & Quade, 1991	588 community health nursing leaders from a national sample	Investigator designed survey based upon NLN and ACHNE criteria	Core content included administration, epidemiology, community health assessment
Towers, 1989; 1990	5964 NPs from a national sample	Investigator designed survey	50% FNPs were master's prepared compared with 24.8% of women's health NPs
Whitfill & Burst, 1994	40 CNM programs	Program description survey	Majority of CNM programs are contained within MS programs

and nonmaster's prepared PNPs. The authors made a case for maintaining both the certificate and master's programs; but ten years later faculty may not want to follow this recommendation unless a certificate program were of a post-master's nature.

Dunn (1993b) reported a more recent national study of PNPs who were members of the National Association of Pediatric Nurse Practitioners (NAPNP). In 1992, 38.5% of those surveyed had been prepared at the master's level as compared with 17% in 1977 (Dunn, 1993a). Regardless of educational preparation, PNPs were providing independent primary care to children in a variety of settings. Most often these children were from low socioeconomic groups (Dunn, 1993b). Thus, faculty do have the data to support the fact that nurse practitioners are meeting the health care needs of underserved groups.

Towers (1989) surveyed 12,000 members of the American Academy of Nurse Practitioners. Almost 50% responded, which is sufficient to evaluate national employment trends. Those with master's degrees ranged from 52.5% for family nurse practitioners to 24.8% for women's health practitioners. More than three-fourths of psychiatric specialists had master's degrees. The majority worked in urban areas and almost one-quarter had hospital admitting privileges (Towers, 1990).

Knowing how current practitioners are used is important because this information can be used to justify program design, including clinical practicums contained therein. Equally important for future planning is employers' willingness to use graduates from nurse practitioner programs. Louis and Sabo (1994) investigated disposition to hire nurse practitioners in Nevada. Study participants included nurse practitioners, nurse executives, and physicians. Less than 25% of mailed surveys were returned; only 43% of physicians had experience with practitioners. Seventy-one percent of physicians and 42% of nursing administrators saw a need for them, and 26% of physicians said they would not hire NPs even though they had had experience with them. Respondents most frequently cited the need for family and gerontological nurse practitioners. Physicians and others with baccalaureate and higher university saw less need for NPs than did those with diplomas and associate degrees. The authors wondered if a master's degree had been required of all NPs, as was not the case, would the responses have been different. Not knowing what the scope of practice for NPs may have been a problem for the survey respondents. One of the major recommendations of the study was to disseminate more information regarding nurse practitioners. What seems clear, then, is that faculty planning nurse practitioner programs need to meet with potential employers and help them understand the role of the nurse practitioner. Reticence to use nurse practitioners may have been related to lack of knowledge about the role.

Assessing the specific need and utilization for clinical specialists was frequently reported by specialty area of practice. For example, Segall and McKay (1984) surveyed community health graduates from one school in Colorado and their supervisors and Selby, Riportell-Muller, Salmon, Lagault, and Quade (1991) sampled community health nursing leaders nationwide.* Segall and McKay (1984) found that 46% of the graduates were employed in education, 39% in administration, and 15% in clinical practice. Graduates rated clinical content as the most useful and functional role content the least beneficial. The authors attributed this finding to the fact that graduates may have had an increased demand for advanced clinical knowledge. Graduates saw the need, however, for additional content in administration. Respondents and their supervisors validated success in the job environment.

Selby's et al. (1991) more recent survey of community health nursing educational needs supported Segall and McKay's (1984) finding that administration and management should be included in community health programs as community health leaders believed the administrator-manager role the most important with direct care roles and beginning competency next. A majority also identified the importance of the researcher and consultant roles. The investigators discovered that while the administration-management role was critical, less than 30% of the master's programs required beginning competency in this area. The researcher role was the only listed educational competency that exceeded practice requirements. Given practice requirements, the authors recommended faculty examine the nature of nursing core courses required of community health graduates. They also said that more emphasis be placed on epidemiological theories. One could also conclude that faculty teaching in community health majors may want to enhance administrative role content and explore what research competencies are required in contradistinction to requirements at the doctoral level.

Included in the plans for health care reform is health care offered at the work site. Occupational health nurses will be critical to that effort. Two nationwide surveys delineated the roles for master's prepared occupational health nurses (Christensen, Richard, Froberg, McGovern & Abanobi, 1985; Guzik, McGovern, & Kochervar, 1992; McGovern, Richard, Christensen, Froberg, & Abanobi, 1985). Most respondents in the 1985 survey were employed in administrative positions and were actively involved in program planning and organizational decision making

---

*Some authors currently do not include community health/public health nurses in the category of advanced nurse practitioners which includes the employment categories of clinical specialists and nurse practitioners (Cronenwett, 1995). However, federal data sets would include this specialization under the rubric of clinical practice if such nurses did not serve in an administrative capacity.

regardless of course preparation in these two area. The other respondents were employed as educators and nurse practitioners (Christensen et al., 1985).

The 1992 study complemented the database regarding occupational health nurses (Guzik & McGovern, 1992). This study described the roles of master's prepared nurses who functioned as both consultants within an employer's firm and those who consulted with companies external to one employer agency. Over three-fourths of the graduates from 10 different schools were actually employed as occupational health nurses in a variety of for profit and nonprofit agencies. Using data from a previous survey (Christensen et al., 1985), the authors estimated that 89% of those master's prepared in occupational health nursing and working in the field responded to their current survey. One strength of the study was that role theory guided the selection of job satisfaction and work situation variables. An extensive table depicted the operationalization of these two variables. Both internal and external consultants expressed moderate satisfaction with their jobs. These occupational health nurses performed similar tasks when compared to those from earlier studies. However, the 1992 respondents were more concerned with environmental issues. Knowledge of environmental issues is an example of the type of information that could be gained through interdisciplinary course work.

Home care is another critical element of the current and future health care delivery system. Barkauskas and Blaha (1989) found no specific master's programs in home care, but 9 programs offered a subspecialty in home care and 10 others offered specific courses.

Mental health clinical specialists also fill important roles within the health care system. Brophy, Rankin, Butler, and Egenes (1989) found that 96% of the hospitals that responded to their survey already employed such specialists. Critical content identified for a master's program included treatment modalities, general nursing knowledge, and administration/management. Respondents perceived teaching and staff development roles essential for the clinical specialists.

Derstine (1992) reported a follow-up study of graduates who majored in rehabilitation nursing. One year following graduation, only 3 of 12 graduates specifically identified themselves as rehabilitation clinical specialists. Others were in fields, such as quality assurance, where they used the rehabilitation content. Some graduates said that even though they didn't intend to be employed in rehabilitation, the content was helpful their jobs. Employers stated graduates were effectively using the program's content and expected graduates to solve problems, improve quality of care, and provide leadership to others. These findings support the notion that a clinical specialist curriculum helps prepare graduates for a variety of roles.

The oncology field is another area that employs clinical specialists. The Oncology Nursing Society (ONS) has been quite active in developing guidelines for master's education (Gallagher, Spross, & Powel, 1992). In preparation for the second Oncology Nurse Specialist (OCNS) conference, Gallagher et al. conducted a two-round Delphi study. Sampling procedures were generally well outlined, but the authors did not specifically report the questionnaire's response rate. Findings revealed that a clinical focus would remain important in the face of a tightened financial environment, with collaboration between clinicians and administrators essential.

Collaboration with administrators is important. Acute care clinical specialists also have felt ill-prepared to deal with administration issues (Radke, McArt, Schmitt, & Walker, 1990). Radke et al. sought to gather data from graduates of one program regarding past, present, and future administrative duties. In graduate school, 21% had taken courses with administration content and 85% stated their graduate program should have included more content in this arena. Although only 15% currently were employed in administrative positions, many others were involved in decisions regarding institutional policies that required an administrative knowledge base.

All of the previous studies delineating requirements for advanced practice have used survey methodology, most often using samples from one school. Fenton (1992) used qualitative methods guided by Benner's (1984) work, to identify competencies displayed by clinical nurse specialists. Observed competencies were: the helping role, administrating and monitoring therapeutic interventions, management of rapidly changing situations, diagnostic and monitoring function, teaching/coaching function, quality assessment functions, and organization and work role competencies necessary to function within a bureaucracy. In addition, a consultation role was identified. Assertive clinical specialists had more effective role performance. Each competency was described in full, but the author provided no direct quotes from study participants. This may have been because this article presented a secondary data analysis of previously reported research. The author concluded that master's curricula for clinical specialists should focus on these identified competencies which were similarly identified by participants in other studies.

Some have proposed that dimensions of the nurse practitioner and clinical specialist roles are similar. Three recent research studies (Elder & Bullough, 1990; Fenton & Brykczynski, 1993; Forbes, Rafson, Spross, & Kozlowski, 1990), as well as a recent presentation to the AACN (Cronenwett, 1995), support this contention. Forbes et al. (1990) conducted a survey of graduate programs in the United States with clinical specialist and/or practitioner programs. Findings revealed that curricula in both kinds of programs were similar; but, practitioner programs contained more physical assessment and history taking, pharmacology, nutrition, and primary care. NP graduates functioned more in primary care and CNSs were in tertiary care settings. The authors suggested that CNS and NP programs might be merged.

Elder and Bullough's (1990) survey of graduates from one nursing program and Fenton and Brykczynski's (1993) study supported Forbes' et al. recommendation. Elder and Bullough (1990) discovered both NPs and CNSs engaged in similar activities. However, NPs did more physical exams and prescribed treatments. CNSs participated more in staff development activities.

Fenton and Brykczynski (1993) conducted a secondary analysis on qualitative data previously collected for the purpose of comparing the NP and the CNS role. Findings from this comparative study showed that in addition to the CNS competencies previously described by Fenton (1992), NPs displayed a competency entitled management of patient health/illness status. Further, CNSs had more role ambiguity. These authors suggested that curricula for NPs and CNSs be developed with a common core but different clinical applications.

Additional advanced clinical roles for master's prepared graduates are the Certified Nurse Anesthetist (CRNA) and Certified Nurse Midwife (CNM). Currently, an estimated 7,400 CNMs exist and of those 2,400 have master's degrees (Health Resources and Services Administration, 1990). The number of CRNAs is approximately 18,600 and 3,100 have master's degrees (Health Resources and Services Administration, 1990). By 1998, all CRNA programs will offer only a master's degree (personnel communication, October 27, 1994).

The master's degree is not projected to be a requirement for midwifery certification; however, 32 of 40 programs award a master's degree. Of those, several offer a choice of a certificate or master's degree, and one program awards a Master's in Public Health (Whitfill & Burst, 1994). If faculty are planning curricula for CNM programs, given the trend, a master's program seems to be a wise choice.

Although the purpose of this review is not to evaluate fully the clinical outcomes observed of NPs and CNSs, brief mention should be made of recent studies that document the effectiveness of these roles because curricula should be designed to promote role performance. For example, Baradell (1994) found that as compared to psychologists, master's prepared psychiatric clinical specialists delivered less costly care of equal quality. Ramsey, Edwards, Lenz, Odom, and Brown (1993) reported that 97% of a systematic sample of 101 clients surveyed via telephone were very satisfied with their care from family nurse practitioners. The authors did not say whether or not master's prepared clinicians delivered the care. Mahoney (1994) discovered when nurse practitioners were compared to physicians on appropriateness of prescribing medications for the elderly, the NPs' practice was more appropriate even though the physicians had more years of experience. Again, no mention was made of the NPs' educational preparation. However, one might assume that current curricula, including those at the master's level, are preparing graduates to meet the needs of patients in primary care settings.

No mention has been made of doctorally prepared clinicians. And, indeed only 7% of all nurses with doctorates listed clinical practice as their primary employment area as compared with 64% of master's prepared nurses (Health Resources and Services Administration, 1994a). Many master's prepared nurses, however, might need further education in order to better function in the current advanced nursing practice roles. Therefore, nursing faculty might consider the development of clinical programs at the post-master's level.

EDUCATOR AND RESEARCHER ROLES

According to Rosenfeld (1993), 11,533 or 69.7% of all nursing faculty have the master's degree as their highest credential; the remaining have doctoral degrees (see Table 6.1). Table 6.5 summarizes studies concerned with those who hold educator roles.

Since most master's programs have a heavy clinical emphasis, how faculty acquire skills for teaching is of some concern. Oermann and Jamison (1989) investigated the extent to which nursing education content was found in master's programs. The data showed that only 10 programs offered a major in nursing education, 34 programs offered minors, 18 programs had electives in nursing education, and 14 had tracks or other curricular designs. Fifteen programs had no nursing education courses. Numbers of credit hours in nursing education ranged from 2 to 20.

Because Canadians have a goal of having the baccalaureate degree for entry into practice by the year 2000, an adequate pool of faculty will be needed. Therefore, Ford and Wertenberger (1993) partially replicated, within the Canadian environment, Oermann and Jamison's study. One strength of their research report was that they included sample questions from the survey in a table. All 10 Canadian master's programs took part in their study. Results showed that dual role preparation was the norm and seven programs offered nursing education courses. Most programs offered 1 to 2 nursing education courses. While the purpose of the courses was to prepare nurse educators, course work appeared to contain just an overview of knowledge and skills required for the teaching role. They suggested more education course work be required, but they could be offered in departments outside nursing. Since most nursing faculty in the United States are prepared at the master's level,

Table 6.5   Educator and Researcher Roles

Author/Date	Sample	Method	Findings
Farren, 1991	National sample of 152 doctorally prepared nurses	Investigator designed descriptive-correlational survey	Employer support, type of degree, and participating in faculty research while a student correlated with current productivity
Ford & Wertenberger, 1993	10 Canadian master's programs	Survey using previously published instrument	7 of 10 programs have nursing education coursework; 2 others require courses outside department
Holzemer, 1987	14 doctoral programs	Investigator designed survey modified from previously published instruments	Between 1979 and 1984 percentage of time faculty devoted to research increased
Holzemer & Chambers, 1986	326 faculty 659 students 296 alumni	Investigator designed survey modified from previously published instruments	Extramural funding was predictive of alumni productivity
Karuhije, 1986	211 nurse educators	Investigator designed survey	Educators felt ill prepared for clinical teaching role
Keck, 1992	133 traditional MS students 152 ITV students	Quasi-experimental with intact groups	Little difference in learning outcomes
Lash, 1987	31 doctoral programs	Perusal of NLN documents	Curricula differed little among various program types
Lash, 1992	255 nurse doctorates from national sample	Investigator designed survey used for path analysis	Graduation from top ranked school an important predictor of career attainment
Lott, Anderson, & Kenner, 1993	11 master's prepared undergraduate faculty members	Interviews analyzed thorough content analysis	Faculty exhibit a variety of feelings and symptoms related to role stress and strain
Megel, Langston, & Creswell, 1988	148 leading nurse researchers	Investigator designed survey	High producers identified with peers outside institution and taught less than low producers

Table 6.5 *Continued*

Author/Date	Sample	Method	Findings
Oermann & Jamison, 1989	92 master's programs	Investigator designed survey	10 programs offered nursing education major. Others had minors, electives, or tracks
Reilly, 1990	One master's program	Case study	Outreach programs are a viable alternative for master's degree programs
Snyder-Halpern, 1986	8 doctoral programs	Case study	PhD and DNSc programs were more alike than different
Zebelman & Olswang, 1989	788 doctoral students from national sample	Investigator designed survey	After first year of study, more students interested in research than teaching

curriculum planners may want to consider Ford and Wertenberger's suggested approach to providing additional course work for potential nurse educators. Combining educational content taught within and outside a college of nursing might be the most efficacious to provide students with the opportunity to learn about educating students within higher education settings.

Investigating coursework required does shed some light on the extensiveness of preparation for the teaching role. However, faculty's perception of the adequacy of their preparation may help curriculum planners consider what might be needed in any curriculum revision. Karuhije (1986) used a convenience sample of educators who had attended an Associate Degree Nursing workshop and faculty who attended a National League for Nursing Convention. Data collection was via a very simple questionnaire which was shown within the article. Seventy-eight percent of survey respondents agreed that their preparation for clinical teaching was inadequate. Essential content identified included clinical teaching strategies and clinical evaluation. When one considers that few graduate programs emphasize the nurse educator role, faculty may want to try and integrate the identified essential content into a variety of course offerings.

Many facets of a master's prepared educator's role can cause stress. Lott, Anderson, and Kenner (1993) used qualitative methods to examine how master's prepared educators who teach in undergraduate programs in universities with doctoral programs cope with their environment. A thorough explanation of the study's methodology and data analysis showed role theory formed the basis of the open-ended questions used in the interviews. Data disclosed faculty felt like second-class citizens and perceived pressure to obtain a doctorate. Faculty viewed workload as inequitable among the undergraduate faculty, but not between graduate and undergraduate faculty. They recognized a variety of symptoms associated with stress. To cope with the stress, faculty recommended more open communication between undergraduate and graduate faculty. They also wanted recognition for the contribution master's prepared faculty make to the college's mission. In order to reduce role strain, the authors recommended that colleges facilitate achieving the doctoral degree by reducing workloads and having faculty develop buddy systems to help cope with stress. Lott's et al. findings would probably be supported by many other faculty employed in schools that have the full range of undergraduate and graduate curricula. However, one wonders if faculty at universities without doctoral programs face the same stressors. To help faculty cope with stressors, perhaps teaching practicums should place more emphasis on the totality of the faculty role, not just the actual teaching component. As a consequence, master's graduates might have a more realistic expectation of this role.

Ketefian (1991) and Fitzpatrick (1991) echoed similar sentiments by calling for doctoral programs to prepare students for all dimensions of the faculty role, even though the research role is stressed in doctoral programs. Nursing doctoral programs award primarily the PhD degree. However, the DNS or DNSc programs do not differ substantially in their content devoted to preparing nurse researchers (Lash, 1987; Snyder-Halpern, 1986).

Dennis (1991) stated that students need exposure to a variety of course work and experiences that will foster research careers. Ketefian (1993) made a strong case for not only methodological courses, but courses supported by substantive knowledge used to answer questions of interest to the discipline of nursing. Zebelman and Olswang (1989) found, from a nationwide survey of students in 35 doctoral programs, that the environment of the doctoral program encourages development of a career in research. After one year of study, students appeared to place greater value on developing research expertise rather than in other areas essential to faculty role performance. The authors commented that the desire for a research career may conflict with the actual demands of the environments where most would be employed.

Scholarly productivity is an expectation of graduates and employing institutions, particularly those with graduate programs. Lia-Hoagberg (1985) compared nursing faculty with doctorates to women in other academic fields employed at eight universities. More non-nurse faculty had research-focused careers and had more publications. Nursing faculty had more administrative functions. One reason for this may have been that these faculty were older and had not had the opportunity to develop their research foci.

Holzemer (1987) found that scholarly productivity of faculty increased from 1979 to 1984 as evidenced by the mean number of publications per faculty. In 1979, the mean was 6.6 and 7.4 in 1984. Although the difference was statistically nonsignificant, faculty devoted a greater percentage of time to research in 1984 at the $p = .01$ level. The number of dissertations supported by extramural funding was somewhat predictive of alumni productivity (Holzemer & Chambers, 1986).

More recently Megel, Langston, and Creswell (1988) surveyed researchers who had been identified as top producers by deans at Research I and II universities and health science centers. Generally, high producers identified more with peers outside their institutions and their research team members. They also desired to conduct research more than teaching when compared to low producers. High producers continued to publish with graduate faculty advisors more than did low producers. One interesting finding, however, was that high producers spent more time on administrative duties than their low-producing peers. A strength of this study was the well-outlined methodology. A shortcoming was the researchers did not use portions of Holzemer's instrumentation, nor was his work referenced.

Farren (1991) also examined faculty scholarly productivity, which was defined as the number of research projects not the number of publications. Like Megel et al., she designed her own survey instrument without reference to previously published tools. She used a stratified random sample to gather data from nurses with various doctorates who were listed in the 1984 *American Nurses Association Directory of Nurses with Doctoral Degrees.* Non-nurse doctorates had a higher response rate (90%) than those with doctorates in nursing whose response rate was 67.5%. Consistent with previous research, approximately two-thirds were employed in educational institutions.

Seventy percent had conducted post-dissertation research, which was a marked increase from other research cited by Farren. Computer experience and participating with faculty in research during their doctoral program had significant correlations with current productivity. Nurses with PhDs and DNSs were more productive than those who held the EdD. Institutional support, such as released time and undefined employer support, also correlated with productivity. Similar to Megel, Langston, and Creswell's (1988) findings, Farren found support from peers outside the employing institution was critical to productivity. Another interesting finding was that 42.8% felt able to conduct independent research, while 53.3% identified they needed some assistance, but were able to find that help.

Lash (1992) investigated variables related to the career attainment of faculty with doctoral degrees in nursing. She used the 1984 ANA directory and lists from the degree granting institutions to identify this sample. A path analysis that described career variables in three stages: predoctorate, first job attainment, and current job attainment was founded on prior research. A significant finding was that graduation from a top-ranked school predicted employment in a like institution. Numbers of publications were positively correlated with the ranking of the current employing institution, current faculty rank, predoctoral teaching experience, but not with predoctoral publications. Another finding of import was that faculty rank for the first job post-graduation was higher for those employed at lower ranked schools. The lower professorial rank persisted for those employed at higher ranked institutions, perhaps reflecting the more competitive environments in those schools. Lash stated that recognition by peers in the form of membership in honoraries and other like activities was also a measure of career attainment. Predoctoral recognition and current publications contributed strongly to the recognition. Lash cautioned that expansion of the numbers of doctoral programs might not be accompanied by an expansion of the quality and quantity of scholarly productivity for nursing as a whole. When her recommendations are considered along with Ketefian's (1991) and Fitzpatrick's (1991) recommendations, doctoral program faculty have further support for the notion that all components of the faculty role need emphasis in doctoral programs. Even though many doctoral candidates may already be experienced in their teaching and service roles, they may need reinforcement for the idea that these roles will not be deemphasized when the research role is added.

NURSING ADMINISTRATORS

An estimated 42,000 nursing administrators hold master's degrees and fewer than 1,000 have doctorates. The percentage of these degrees is in nursing is unknown (Health Resources and Human Services Administration, 1994a). Knowing what knowledge and skills are needed for these administrators seems particularly important if graduates are to serve as leaders in a turbulent health care system. The number of articles in the literature, however, which could be used in curriculum planning were much lower than those available for the clinical and educator roles (see Table 6.6).

Price (1984) surveyed graduates from master's programs with a major or functional component in nursing administration and their employers. A nursing administration program evaluation instrument was modified for use in her study.

Table 6.6   Nurse Administrators

Author/Date	Sample	Method	Findings
Minnick, 1993	279 MSN students 57 MSN/MBA dual degree students 23 other students	Investigator designed survey	Dual degree students more likely to seek jobs outside hospital. Dual degree programs may keep students within nursing
Price, 1984	10 nursing administration master's programs	Survey using previously published instrument	Described overview of curricula
Smith, T., 1993	75 directors of nursing	Investigator designed survey	Needed skills included conceptual, human, and technical
Wagner, Henry, Giovinco, & Blanks, 1988	37 publications	Content Analysis	Important content areas included health policy, nursing practice, research, and finance

Over 50% of graduates expressed satisfaction with their education. Graduates from programs with solely an administrative focus thought their education contributed more to the effectiveness of their leadership skills than did graduates from other programs. No relationship existed between the level of graduates' perceived attainment of program goals and employer satisfaction with the graduates' performance. Graduates wanted more content in the area of financial management and, for the most part, did not perceive the need for advanced clinical knowledge.

Wagner, Henry, Giovinco, and Blanks (1988) analyzed 37 publications from the years 1976–1985 for recommendations regarding content for master's programs in nursing administration. They thoroughly described the content analysis and interrater reliability procedures. Data showed that content fell into the domains of organizational systems, political environment, economic concerns, and accounting and cost procedures. In addition, human resource management and work redesign seemed important. Twenty articles made mention of nursing theoretical foundations, but only two referred to clinical specialization. Their findings seem to support content identified as relevant by the respondents in Price's (1984) study.

Minnick (1993) contacted students enrolled in master's degree programs in nursing administration, dual MBA/MSN programs, as well as students in a variety of other dual-degree programs. She chose the single-focus programs sampled according to similar geographic distribution and academic ratings as compared to the dual-degree programs.

Several findings of note emerged. Dual-degree students were more likely to study full time and seek employment outside a hospital setting. Some of these students stated that they would have attended MBA programs only if a dual-degree program would not have been available. The author postulated that the brightest students may be attracted to these dual-degree programs as their scores on the GRE were higher than MSN students. In other words, these bright students may have been lost to nursing if the dual-degree program had not been available. Given this finding, nursing graduate faculties might want to consider how to incorporate more administrative content into their programs in order to attract these bright students.

The previous studies concentrated, for the most part, on student and graduate perceptions of needed content and skills. Smith (1993), however, explored important skills for effective management from the perspective of the manager. Using a theoretical model derived from Katz (1974), the investigator constructed a reliable and valid survey tool that she sent to a stratified random sample of directors of nursing (presumably the chief nurse executive) at member hospitals of the College of Teaching Hospitals. She placed questionnaire items shown within tables in the article into the categories of conceptual, human, and technical skills. Directors acknowledged the importance of conceptual skills such as analyzing the political dimensions of the work environment and designing and implementing organizational structure; but, they saw a need for improved performance in these areas. Directors said human skills such as interpersonal communication needed improvement and rated skills in this domain as highly important for effective performance. Only 18.3% of the directors reported conflicting expectations of the educational program and job requirements with regard to technical skills such as financial management. For all skill dimensions, a positive correlation existed between self-assessment and importance of skill behaviors. These skill dimensions were similar in nature to those identified by Price (1984) and Wagner et al., (1988).

One trend noted in the studies concerned with the nursing administrator role is the fact that many of the skills are of an interdisciplinary nature. And, administrators have to, on a daily basis, work within an interdisciplinary environment. Therefore, faculty may want to consider locating some coursework or potential administrators in an interdisciplinary environment.

SUMMARY

A voluminous amount of research exists regarding the utilization of graduates from master's and doctoral programs. With the exception of national data sets from the federal government and national surveys sponsored by professional organizations, most authors have conducted local studies of master's graduates. Studies of doctoral programs were more national in scope, perhaps because the target population was smaller.

Data were gathered primarily through investigator-designed instruments and study conclusions were drawn mainly from descriptive-correlational statistics. Lash's (1992) study was a notable exception. Studying utilization and effectiveness of nurses in advanced clinical practice, however, was amenable to other means as evidenced by Fenton and Brykczynski's (1993) work.

Despite the fact that many of the studies were limited in scope, a consensus of findings seemed to emerge. Graduates from master's programs and their employers want nurses who can function in a multiplicity of roles. Both clinical nurse specialists and nurse practitioners need to have a core of advanced nursing knowledge which will allow them to function in a variety of settings. The demand for clinical knowledge has remained stable over time, but acquisition of such knowledge is not sufficient for effective role performance. Most advanced nurse practitioners need some administrative skills and knowledge to function competently in the complex organizations in which they work. Administrators, on the other hand, may need more knowledge and skills in the administrative arena and less in the clinical.

Most doctoral program graduates work in academic institutions which place multiple demands on their time. Many graduates had the expectation that research would be a priority in their careers. However, with the exception of those in top-ranked universities, teaching may take a higher priority. For those educators with a master's degree, role confusion, stress, and strain will continue as they try to compete with doctorally prepared faculty.

FUTURE DIRECTIONS

Anticipating how nursing curricula should be changed in order to prepare graduates for an ever-changing health care system is challenging to say the least. A *Report to Congress* (Health Resources and Services Administration, 1990), states that the need for those with master's and doctoral degrees will grow. While the total of nurses with master's degrees is estimated to be 240,000, the projected demand is for 363,000. Not only will the numbers of graduates have to increase, but educators will have to find innovative ways to educate students who can be flexible in meeting the needs of the health care system. One report suggests that an argument against required master's preparation for nurse practitioners is lack of available programs in rural and underserved areas (Fowkes, Gamel, Garcia, Wilson, & Stewart, 1993). But, distance learning strategies could be used for students in these geographic areas without compromising quality (Keck, 1992; Reilly, 1990).

Changing demographics will necessitate curricula that address the needs of the elderly in primary and long-term care settings. Health care system complexity will also require graduates who have excellent communication skills in order for them to function effectively in interdisciplinary environments (Lenz, 1994).

As the need for master's graduates increases, a concomitant need for doctorally prepared faculty will increase. Full-time faculty line vacancies have been fairly stable for the past several years (Rosenfeld, 1993). The increased use of part-time faculty and perhaps the lack of qualified full-time faculty has caused some universities to recapture the nursing lines and reallocate them to other departments. However, as current faculty retire, the need for faculty may further outstrip the supply. Therefore, doctoral program faculty will have to find ways to educate students who cannot attend school full time. Outreach, weekend, and summer programs may need to become the norm. In that environment, mentoring students in a way to foster their research careers will be challenging.

Providing master's and doctoral programs that use flexible teaching/learning strategies will not be enough. Nursing faculty will have to have a constant sense of what skills and knowledge are needed to function in an uncertain environment. To that end, local follow-up studies of graduates and their employers may give useful information. However, larger cross-institutional studies may better facilitate local, state, regional, and federal planning. Institutions could share data collection instruments rather than each evaluation team developing its own. Thus, data could be pooled and compared. Studies using qualitative methodologies could assist faculty in better understanding the nuances of advanced practice so that they could better incorporate the realities of the practice environment into their educational programs.

Finally, the research suggests that the most productive, in terms of scholarship, doctorally prepared faculty are concentrated in the top ranked schools. Given the available funding resources, this pattern is likely to continue. However, a need will continue to exist for doctoral education outside the top ranked schools. Perhaps those schools should prepare students who can meet the demands of faculty roles in places which are not centers of research excellence, but do provide top quality undergraduate and graduate education. Those faculty whose primary emphasis is teaching might focus their scholarship in the areas of advanced clinical practice; and they might conduct research in partnerships with the major university settings. Talent exists nationwide. Multi-institution collaboration will help capture that talent and advance the discipline of nursing.

Graduate programs have a vital role to play in providing education for advanced nurse practitioners, faculty, researchers, and administrators. Continued research concerned with the utilization and effectiveness of the graduates will help faculty to improve current curricula and to plan for the future health care system.

REFERENCES

American Nurses Association. (1984). *Directory of nurses with doctoral degrees* (Publication No. G-143). Kansas City, MO: Author.

American Nurses Association. (1992). *Nursing's agenda for health care reform* (Publication No. PR-3). Washington, DC: Author.

Baradell, J. G. (1994). Cost-effectiveness and quality of care provided by clinical nurse specialists. *Journal of Psychosocial Nursing, 32*(3), 21–24.

Barkauskas, V. H., & Blaha, A. J. (1989). A survey of home care programs. *Caring, 8*(2), 16–20.

Benner, P. (1984). *From novice to expert.* Menlo Park, CA: Addison-Wesley.

Brimmer, P. F., Skoner, M. M., Pender, N. J., Williams, C. A., Fleming, J. W., & Werley, H. H. (1983). Nurses with doctoral degrees: Education and employment characteristics. *Research in Nursing and Health, 6,* 157–165.

Brophy, E. B., Rankin, D., Butler, S., & Egenes, K. (1989). The master's prepared mental health nurse: An assessment of employer expectations. *Journal of Nursing Education, 28,* 156–160.

Brown, J. M. (1978). Master's education in nursing, 1945–1969. In M. Louise Fitzpatrick (Ed.), *Historical studies in nursing* (pp. 104–130). New York: Teachers College Press.

Burns, P. G., Nishikawa, H. A., Weatherby, F., Forni, P. R., Moran, M., & Allen, M. E. (1993). Master's degree nursing education: State of the art. *Journal of Professional Nursing, 9,* 267–277.

Christensen, M., Richard, E., Froberg, D., McGovern, P., & Abanobi, O. C. (1985). An analysis of the employment patterns, roles, and functions of master's prepared occupational health nurses; Part II. *Occupational Health Nursing, 33,* 453–459.

Cronenwett, L. (1995). Molding the future for advanced practice nurses: Education, regulation, and practice. In *Role Differentiation of the Nurse Practitioner and Clinical Nurse Specialist: Reaching Toward Consensus* (pp. 1–20). Washington, DC: American Association of Colleges of Nursing.

172 Betsy Frank

Cruikshank, B. M., & Lakin, J. A. (1986). Professional and employment characteristics of NPs with master's preparation and non-master's preparation. *Nurse Practitioner, 11*(11), 45–52.

Dennis, K. E. (1991). Components of the doctoral curriculum that build success in the clinical nurse researcher role. *Journal of Professional Education, 7,* 160–165.

Derstine, J. B. (1992). The rehabilitation clinical nurse specialist of the 1990s: Roles assumed by recent graduates. *Rehabilitation Nursing, 17,* 139–140.

Dunn, A. M. (1993a). 1992 NAPNAP membership survey part I: Member characteristics, issues, and opinions. *Journal of Pediatric Health Care, 7,* 245–250.

Dunn, A. M. (1993b). 1992 NAPNAP membership survey part II: Practice characteristics of pediatric nurse practitioners indicate greater autonomy for PNPs. *Journal of Pediatric Health Care, 7,* 296–302.

Elder, R. G., & Bullough, B. (1990). Nurse practitioners and clinical specialists: Are the roles merging? *Clinical Nurse Specialist, 4*(2), 78–84.

Farren, E. A. (1991). Doctoral preparation and research productivity. *Nursing Outlook, 39,* 22–25.

Fenton, M. V. (1992). Education for the advanced practice of clinical nurse specialists. *Oncology Nursing Forum, 19* (Suppl. 1), 16–20.

Fenton, M. V., & Brykczynski, K. A. (1993). Qualitative distinctions and similarities in the practice of clinical nurse specialists and nurse practitioners. *Journal of Professional Nursing, 9,* 313–326.

Fitzpatrick, M. L. (1991). Doctoral preparation versus expectations. *Journal of Professional Nursing, 7,* 172–176.

Forbes, K. E., Rafson, J., Spross, J. A., & Kozlowski, D. (1990). Clinical nurse specialist and nurse practitioner core curricula survey results. *Nurse Practitioner, 17*(4), 43–48.

Ford, J. S., & Wertenberger, D. H. (1993). Nursing education content in master's in nursing programs. *Canadian Journal of Nursing Education, 25*(2), 53–61.

Fowkes, V., Gamel, N. N., Garcia, R. D., Wilson, S. R., & Stewart, B. R. (1993). *Assessment of physician assistant (PA), nurse practitioner (NP), and nurse-midwife (CNM) training on meeting health-care needs of the underserved* (Contract No. 240-91-0050). Rockville, MD: Office of Program Development, Bureau of Health Professions.

Gallagher, J., Spross, J. A., & Powel, L. L. (1992). Introduction and overview of the conference. *Oncology Nursing Forum* (Suppl. 1), 7–10.

Guzik, V. L., McGovern, P. M., & Kochervar, L. K. (1992). Role function and job satisfaction. *AAOHN Journal, 40,* 521–530.

Health Resources and Services Administration. (1990). *Report to congress on the study of need for nurse advanced trained specialists* (NTIS No. PB 91-105155).

Health Resources and Services Administration. (1994a). *The registered nurse population: Findings from the national sample survey of registered nurses, March, 1992* (ISBN 0-16-042616-2). Washington, DC: US Government Printing Office.

Health Resources and Services Administration. (1994b). *Survey of certified nurse practitioners and clinical nurse specialists: December 1992* (NTIS No. PB 94-158169).

Heller, B. R., Damrosch, S. P., Romano, C. A., & McCarthy, M. R. (1989). Graduate specialization in nursing informatics. *Computers in Nursing, 7,* 68–76.

Hill, B. A. (1989). The development of a master's degree program based on perceived future needs. *Journal of Nursing Education, 28,* 307–313.

Holzemer, W. L. (1987). Doctoral education in nursing: An assessment in quality, 1979–1984. *Nursing Research, 36,* 111–116.

Holzemer, W. L., & Chambers, D. B. (1986). Healthy doctoral programs: Relationship between perceptions of the academic environment and productivity of faculty and alumni. *Research in Nursing and Health, 9,* 299–307.

Hudacek, S., & Carpenter, D. M. (1994). Doctoral education in nursing: A comprehensive review of the research and theoretical literature. In L. R. Allen (Ed.), *Review of research in nursing education* (pp. 57–90). New York: National League for Nursing Press.

Hungler, B. P., Krawczyk, R., Joyce, A., & Polit, D. (1979). *Journal of Advanced Nursing, 4,* 193–203.

Katz, R. L. (1974). Skills of an effective administrator. *Harvard Business Review, 52,* 90–102.

Karuhije, H. F. (1986). Educational preparation for clinical teaching: Perceptions of nurse educators. *Journal of Nursing Education, 25,* 137–144.

Keck, J. F. (1992). Comparison of learning outcomes between graduate students in telecourses and those in traditional classrooms. *Journal of Nursing Education, 31,* 229–234.

Ketefian, S. (1991). Doctoral preparation for faculty roles: Expectations and realities. *Journal of Professional Nursing, 7,* 105–111.

Ketefian, S. (1993). Essentials of doctoral education: Organization of program around knowledge areas. *Journal of Professional Nursing, 9,* 255–261.

Lash, A. A. (1987). Rival conceptions in doctoral education in nursing and their outcomes: An update. *Journal of Nursing Education, 26,* 221–227.

Lash, A. A. (1992). Determinants of career attainments of doctorates in nursing. *Nursing Research, 41,* 216–222.

Lenz, E. R. (1994). *Paradigm shifts, changing contexts, and graduate nursing education.* In J. Kelley (ed.), *A changing health care system* (pp. 19–22). Atlanta: Southern Council for Collegiate Education in Nursing.

Lia-Hoagberg, B. (1985). Comparison of professional activities of nurse doctorates and other academic women. *Nursing Research, 34,* 155–159.

Lott, J. W., Anderson, E. R., & Kenner, C. (1993). Role stress and strain among nondoctorally prepared undergraduate faculty in a school of nursing with a doctoral program. *Journal of Professional Nursing, 9,* 14–22.

Louis, M., & Sabo, C. E. (1994). Nurse practitioners: Need for and willingness to hire as viewed by nurse administrators, nurse practitioners, and physicians. *Journal of the American Academy of Nurse Practitioners, 6,* 113–119.

Mahoney, D. F. (1994). The appropriateness of geriatric prescribing decisions made by nurse practitioners and physicians. *Image: The Journal of Nursing Scholarship, 26,* 41–46.

McGovern, P., Richard, E., Christensen, M., Froberg, D., & Abanobi, O. C. (1985). An analysis of the employment patterns, roles and functions of master's prepared occupational health nurses—Part I. *Occupational Health Nursing, 33,* 407–413.

McLane, A. M. (1978). Core competencies of masters-prepared nurses, *Nursing Research. 27,* 48–53.

Megel, M. E., Langston, N. F., & Creswell, J. W. (1988). Scholarly productivity: A survey of nursing faculty researchers. *Journal of Professional Nursing, 4,* 45–54.

Minnick, A. (1993). MSN in nursing administration and the dual degree. *Nursing and Health Care, 14,* 22–26.

Oermann, M. H., & Jamison, M. T. (1989). Nursing education component in master's programs. *Journal of Nursing Education, 28,* 252–255.

Price, S. A. (1984). Master's programs preparing nursing administrators: What are the essential components? *Journal of Nursing Administration, 14*(1), 11–17.

Radke, K., McArt, E., Schmitt, M., & Walker, E. K. (1990). Administrative preparation of clinical nurse specialists. *Journal of Professional Nursing, 6,* 221–228.

Ramsey, P., Edwards, J., Lenz, C., Odom, J. E., & Brown, B. (1993). Types of health problems and satisfaction with services in a rural nurse-managed clinic. *Journal of Community Health Nursing, 10,* 161–170.

Reilly, D. E. (1990). *Graduate professional education through outreach: A nursing case study.* New York: National League for Nursing Press.

Rosenfeld, P. (1993). *Nurse educators 1993: Findings from the faculty census.* New York: National League for Nursing.

Segall, M., & McKay, R. (1984). Evolution of an aggregate-based community health curriculum. *Nursing Outlook, 32,* 308–312.

Selby, M. L., Riportella-Muller, R., Salmon, M. E., Legault, C., & Quade, D. (1991). Master's degree-level community health nursing educational needs: A national survey of leaders on service and education. *Journal of Professional Nursing, 7,* 88–98.

Smith, M. C. (1980). Evaluation of master's program by graduates and their employers. *Journal of Nursing Education, 19*(9), 4–10.

Smith, T. (1993). Management skills for directors of nursing. *Journal of Nursing Administration, 23*(9), 38–49.

Snyder-Halpern, R. (1986). Doctoral programs in nursing: An examination of curriculum similarities and differences. *Journal of Nursing Education, 25,* 359–365.

Towers, J. (1989). Part I report of the American Academy of Nurse Practitioners' national nurse practitioner survey. *Journal of the American Academy of Nurse Practitioners, 1,* 91–94.

Towers, J. (1990). Report of the national survey of the American academy of nurse practitioners, Part IV: Practice characteristics and marketing activities of nurse practitioners. *Journal of the American Academy of Nurse Practitioners, 2,* 164–167.

Wagner, L., Henry, B., Giovinco, G., & Blanks, C. (1988). Suggestions for graduate education in nursing service administration. *Journal of Nursing Education, 27,* 210–218.

Whitfill, K. A., & Burst, H. V. (1994). ACNM accredited and pre-accredited nurse-midwifery education programs: Program information. *Journal of Nurse Midwifery, 39,* 221–236.

Zebelman, E. S., & Olswang, S. G. (1989). Student career goal changes during doctoral education in nursing. *Journal of Nursing Education, 28,* 53–60.

Chapter Seven

PREDICTING SUCCESS ON THE REGISTERED NURSE LICENSURE EXAMINATION: PAST, PRESENT, AND FUTURE

Dona Rinaldi Carpenter, EdD, RN
Patricia Bailey, EdD, RN

Nurse educators have repeatedly examined factors related to success on the Registered Nurse (RN) Licensure examination, searching for the variable or combination of variables that best predict a student's probability to succeed on the examination. Educators have a responsibility to prepare graduates capable of ensuring minimal public safety in their professional practice. Preparing students to take the RN licensure examination is one mechanism to evaluate whether or not students have attained minimum competency to ensure safe practice.

This review presents the findings of published research addressing predictors of success on the NCLEX-RN examination from 1976 to 1995. To provide a context, a brief history of licensure precedes the literature review. Sixty-two studies published from 1976 through 1995 were included. Table 7.1 highlights the purpose, predictor variables, statistical methods, and findings for each study reviewed. For a review of literature related to predictors of success on the RN Licensure examination prior to 1976, see Taylor, Nahm, Quinn, Harms, Mulaik, and Mulaik (1965), Taylor, Nahm, Loy, Harms, Berthod, and Wolfer (1966), and Schwirian, Baer, Basta, and Larabee (1978).

A computerized search was conducted utilizing the Cumulative Index to Nursing and Allied Literature CD-ROM in addition to extending the search through indexes and references. The general topic searched was "predictors of success on the NCLEX-RN" (National Council Licensure Examinations—Registered Nurse). Subtopics searched included program type (diploma, associate, and baccalaureate), NCLEX structure and validity, minority students, academic and nonacademic variables, and curricular issues (integration, acceleration, upper division). Dissertation Abstracts International was also utilized to gather data from scholars'

Table 7.1 Chronological Summary of Predictor Variables Examined in the Research Literature from 1976–1994

Author	Date	Purpose	Sample	Predictor Variables	Statistical Methods	Findings
Bell, J. A., & Martindill, C. F.	1976	To derive prediction equations for each of the five licensure examinations and to cross-validate the predictors with an independent sample of students.	101 nursing students that graduated from a baccalaureate program in Houston Texas. Second sample of nurses from the same school who graduated a year later were used to cross-validate the prediction equations	NLN achievement tests: Medical Surgical I, Medical Surgical II, Nursing of children, Obstetric Nursing, Psychiatric Nursing	Stepwise regression analysis, cross validation correlations ($p < .01–.05$)	NLN test scores in Nursing of Children and Obstetric Nursing were consistently the best indicators of performance on the SBE's. The results suggest that nursing programs should develop and validate prediction equations to assist nurses in preparing for SBE's
Deardorff, M., Denner, P., & Miller, C.	1976	To develop and validate empirically equations for predicting SBE scores of graduates of an associate degree nursing program from performance on NLN achievement tests	Graduates of a midwestern associate degree nursing program 1969–1974	NLN achievement tests were used: Medical Nursing, Surgical Nursing, Nursing Practice, Facts and Principles, Antepartum Postpartum, Newborn Growth, and Development, Sick Children	Multiple regression, correlation ($p < .05$)	For associate degree nursing students selected sets of National League for Nursing achievement test scores were found to be effective predictors of state board examination scores

(Continued)

Table 7.1 *(Continued)*

Author	Date	Purpose	Sample	Predictor Variables	Statistical Methods	Findings
Perez, T. L.	1977	To develop regression analysis equations for predicting State Board Examination scores of applicants to the nursing major using predictor variables available at the completion of the sophomore year of a baccalaureate program in nursing	B.S.N. graduates of a private liberal arts college, 1968–1977	American College Testing Scores (ACT) G.P.A.'s at various academic levels G.P.A.'s for science and social science courses and an NLN exam score	Multiple regression analysis (p < .01–.05).	The discussion suggests that reading ability be investigated as a measure of potential success on State Board Examinations. The ACT social Science Reading Score, G.P.A. upon completion of the freshman year and the G.P.A. for courses in prerequisite social sciences emerged as the most sensitive predictors of success
Outtz, J. H.	1979	To establish predictors of success on SBTPE for blacks	110 black nursing students who graduated from a baccalaureate program between 1973–1977	Cumulative GPA in High School and College GPA in High School science and math courses GPA in college science courses SAT: Verbal and Math Total	Stepwise multiple regression, Pearson product moment correlation (p < .01–05)	SAT scores were found to be significantly correlated with SBTPE. Positive relationship between high school GPA and College GPA. Positive relationship between high school science and college science grades. Cumulative GPA in college via multiple regression analysis showed as best predictor of success
Washburn, J.	1980	To discover the relationship between NLN Achievement Test Scores and State Board Performance	166 graduates of a diploma degree School of Nursing between 1976 and 1978	Nursing Care of Patients, 1, 2, 3	Pearson product correlation (p < .01)	NLN Achievement test scores had a highly significant correlation with SBTPE result. Nursing Care of Patients II was the best predictor of success. OB NLN achievement test had highest predictor of success on Psychiatric section of SBTPE

Author	Year	Purpose	Sample	Variables	Statistical Analysis	Findings
Melcolm, N., & Bausell, R. B.	1981	To see the degree to which the integrated curriculum influences licensure success	390 baccalaureate graduates of the 1976 and 1977 classes at the University of Maryland School of Nursing	NLN Achievement Scores GPA Individual Grades from Nursing Courses	Simple correlation, forward stepwise multiple regression ($p < .01–.05$)	NLN achievement scores remain good predictors of success on STBPE
Sister St. Thomas	1982	To analyze the relationship between the first semester GPA and the State Board Scores of Vermont College graduates with the ultimate goal of requiring a 1.75 QPI to continue in the nursing major	108 Freshmen nursing students	Freshmen GPA's State Board Scores	Linear regression analysis and pearson product moment ($p < .01–.05$)	Although a significant relationship exists between GPA and nursing board scores a GPA of 1.75 failed to predict success in the state board examination
Aldag, J., & Rose, S.	1983	To determine the relationship between age and American College Testing (ACT) Scores to College GPA and State Board Scores	787 persons admitted to an Associate Degree Program over a 10 year period	Age ACT Scores College GPA and State Board Scores	Pearson product moment ($p < .01$)	More older students passed state board. Age and ACT scores were not correlated with GPA. Age and ACT score were positively correlated with State Board Scores

(Continued)

179

Table 7.1 *Continued*

Author	Date	Purpose	Sample	Predictor Variables	Statistical Methods	Findings
Breyer, F. J.	1984	To assess the ability of the 1982 edition of the Comprehensive Nursing Achievement Test to predict score on NCLEX-RN and to present equations that could predict NCLEX-RN score from the clinical content advisory sub-scores reporte in the 1983 edition of the Comprehensive Nursing Achievement Test	2496 associate degree and diploma students	Comprehensive Nursing Achievement Test	Pearson product moment, multiple regression ($p < .001$)	Strong relationship between success on the Comprehensive Nursing Achievement Test and Success on the RN Licensure Examination
Dell, M. A., & Halpin, G.	1984	To determine which variables were best for predicting program success on State Board Examinations in a predominantly black baccalaureate nursing program	456 black students attending a predominantly black, baccalaureate school of nursing from 1970 to 1974	SAT—Verbal Scores SAT—Quantitative Scores GPA—High School NLN Pre-Nursing	Discriminate Analysis ($p < .001–.05$)	Discriminant analysis showed that the measures significantly differentiated between dropouts and graduates
Sharp, T. G.	1984	To determine whether any one of seven selected variables or a combination of variables is predictive of performance on the State Board Test Pool Examination	322 graduates of The University of Tennessee between 1974 and 1979	High School GPA University GPA ACT Scores [English, Mathematics, Social Studies, Natural Sciences, Composite]	Discriminate analysis, stepwise multiple regression ($p < .0001$)	The variables selected were each found to be predictive of SBTPE performance. The strongest combination for predicting SBTPE performance was found to be GPA, math and natural science ACT scores.

Author	Year	Purpose	Sample	Variables	Analysis	Findings
Yocom, C. J., & Scherubel, J. C.	1985	To examine student performance prior to and following admission to a baccalaureate nursing program in comparison with their performance on the individual sections of the State Board Test Pool Examinations (SBE) and an overall assessment of Pass-Fail on the SBE	139 class of 1980 graduates	Pre-admission GPA's Individual Course Grades Cumulative GPA's for work completed following admission Race The school from which the greatest number of prerequisite courses were completed Previous academic degrees Number of credit hours earned prior to admission	Stepwise multiple regression, Pearson Product Moment Correlation ($p < .001-.05$)	Junior and senior year cumulative clinical nursing theory GPA had the highest weighting for pass/fail on SBE. Clinical nursing theory GPA's were more highly correlated with SBE performance than the clinical nursing practicum
Quick, M. M., Krupa, K. C., & Whitley, T. W.	1985	To determine whether admission data can be used to predict success on the NCLEX-RN in a Baccalaureate Program	182 students who received baccalaureate degrees in 1982, 1983, and 1984	GPA end of Freshman year SAT Verbal Scores Anatomy and physiology grades	Discriminant analysis ($p < .0001$)	Data available at the time of admission to the first clinical nursing course permit prediction of NCLEX-RN performance

(Continued)

181

Table 7.1 *Continued*

Author	Date	Purpose	Sample	Predictor Variables	Statistical Methods	Findings
Felts, J.	1986	To determine which cognitive variables best predict success in nursing courses, and to examine the relationship between selected cognitive variables and performance on the NCLEX-RN	297 first time writers of the NCLEX-RN between July 1992 and February 1984	High School GPA ACT Scores Age Behavioral or Social Science Courses Biological Science Courses Humanities Courses Nursing Courses Physical Science Courses Support Courses Cumulative GPA	Discriminant Analysis and Chi Square (p. < .001).	ACT composite score was found to be the best admission criteria predictor for success in nursing courses with support course GPA and microbiology best predicting overall success in college. Performance in college courses predicted success on the NCLEX-RN with greater accuracy than high school performance. Grades in the biological and social sciences along with humanities differentiate students that pass or fail. The role of nursing courses in relation to the NCLEX-RN was not identified in this study
Glick, O., McClelland, E., & Yang, J.	1986	To investigate the relationship between admission selection variables and subsequent achievement in a baccalaureate program and on the NCLEX-RN; extent to which achievement in clinical courses predicts performance on NCLEX; and relationship among predictor variables	51 graduates, 96% female	Admission selection variables Pre-nursing courses Required Clinical Nursing Courses	Correlation Coefficients, Stepwise multiple regression (p < .001–.05)	When GPA in nursing courses was used as criterion of success, the pre-nursing GPA and Biology GPA correlated most highly. Statistically significant correlations observed among the predictor variables supported the validity of using academic achievement data as selection criteria for admission to a baccalaureate nursing program

Author	Year	Purpose	Sample	Variables	Analysis	Findings
Woodham, R., & Taube, K.	1986	Ex Post Facto correlational study to determine the relationship of selected admission criteria and performance in the integrated nursing major didactic courses of an associate science in nursing degree program as predictors for performance on the licensing examination for registered nurses	104 associate degree nursing graduates	Seven required Associate Degree Nursing Courses SAT verbal scores Age at graduation High school class rank SAT math scores	Pearson Correlation, Multivariate Regression ($p < .01$)	A significant positive relationship was demonstrated with the seven nursing courses and SAT verbal scores. Age at graduation, high school class rank and SAT math scores were not significant in predicting NCLEX performance
Bauwens, E. E., & Gerhard, G. G.	1987	To investigate the Watson-Glaser Critical Thinking Appraisal as a potential predictor of success on NCLEX	177 baccalaureate nursing students who graduated between December 1982 and May 1984	University GPA/Watson Glaser	Pearson Product Moment and Stepwise Multiple Regression ($p < .01–.005$)	Watson Glaser is not a valid measure of specific cognitive processes underlying the nursing process. The usefulness of the Watson-Glaser Critical Thinking Appraisal is in its ability to predict nursing success on a preadmission basis

(Continued)

183

Table 7.1 *Continued*

Author	Date	Purpose	Sample	Predictor Variables	Statistical Methods	Findings
Crane, P., Wright, C. R., & Michael, W. B.	1987	The three major purposes of this investigation were to determine for a total sample of 418 students the validity coefficients of selected predictor variables obtained prior to admission to the program and of eight intermediate variables reflecting scores on standardized achievement tests administered at the conclusion of each of eight courses or course sequences; to ascertain validity coefficients for the same predictors and intermediate variables for each of four ethnic groups; and to identify through the use of multiple regression analyses the combination of two or three predictor variable more prognostic of success	The records of 418 graduating nursing students who had completed a diploma nursing program between the years of 1984 and 1985	Chronological Age Anatomy GPA Physiology GPA Psychology GPA Prerequisite Total GPA California Achievement Tests Reading Comprehension Reading Total Mathematics Concepts and Applications Mathematics Total Anatomy and Physiology Normal Nutrition NLN Fundamentals of Drug Therapy NLN Psychiatric Nursing NLN Nursing the Child-bearing Family NLN Nursing of Children	Correlation, Multiple Regression ($p < .001 - .05$)	Senior GPA is a highly valid predictor of NCLEX-RN scores for members of the White and Hispanic subgroups but only modestly valid for Black and Asian subgroups. High School GPA affords little, if any predictive validity of either criterion measure for any ethnic group. Prerequisite course work taken primarily in a community college affords moderate predictive validity for White, Hispanic, and Asian subgroups but high validity for the black subgroup, in the prediction of Senior GPA but reduced if not marginal validity for all ethnic

Author	Year	Purpose	Sample	Variables	Analysis	Findings
Gross, Y. T., Takazawa, E. S., & Rose, C. L.	1987	To evaluate the impact of the nursing curriculum on the students ability to think critically and to examine the relationship between performance on the Watson-Glaser Critical Thinking appraisal and the NLN preadmission test to GPA and NCLEX	108 associate and baccalaureate students	Age Years of school after high school Ethnicity Watson-Glaser at Entry Watson-Glaser at Exit	Correlations, Multiple Regression (p < .01–.05)	Nursing education improves critical thinking skills and the GPA is more important that the Watson-Glaser in predicting NCLEX performance
Yang, J. C., Glick, O. J., & McClelland, E.	1987	The purpose of this study was to (1) investigate the relationship between admission selection variables and subsequent achievement in an integrated baccalaureate nursing program and performance on the NCLEX-RN; (2) Extent to which achievement in clinical nursing courses predicted performance on the NCLEX RN; (3) Relationship among predictor variables	210 graduates of a baccalaureate nursing program who graduated in 1983, 1984, 1985	High School Record Cumulative Nursing GPA Individual and Composite College Admission Test Scores (ACT) Grades from all required pre-nursing and clinical nursing courses Cumulative GPA for chemistry, biology, and microbiology	Pearson Product Moment Correlation, Stepwise Multiple Regression (p < .01–.05)	When PN-GPA was selected as the criterion of success, PN-GPA and BIO-GPA exhibited the highest correlation coefficients among other predictors for all nursing courses. Although there were high correlations among criterion variables and NCLEX RN scores, none of the predictors showing high correlations were significant predictors of performance on NCLEX-RN. One nursing course (Nursing III) made a significant contribution to the NCLEX scores over and above all other clinical nursing courses.

(Continued)

185

Table 7.1 *Continued*

Author	Date	Purpose	Sample	Predictor Variables	Statistical Methods	Findings
Friedemann, M. L., & Valentine, S.	1988	To further explore pre-nursing student factors and their relationship to success in the licensure examination	164 graduates from 1978–1984 taking the old state board exam, and 159 taking the new examination	Age Number of academic credits completed prior to entering nursing Entry GPA Grades in inorganic or organic chemistry Grades in the program courses consisting of six nursing courses, nutrition, and pharmacology Exit GPA	Anova, Stepwise Multiple Regression ($p < .001–.05$)	Grade point average and student age were most useful in predicting exam scores from the pre-admission variables. Students who received A-grades in lecture courses scored relatively higher and B-Students scored lower on the new licensure examination compared to the old examinations. Students entering the program as LPNs did markedly better on the new licensure examination than they did on the old examinations
Krupa, K. C., Quick, M. M., & Whitley, T. W.	1988	To determine whether grades in nursing courses required of all students could predict National Council Licensure Examination for Registered Nurse performance	The records of 384 nursing students who graduated from a BSN program and took the NCLEX-RN during 1982 through 1985	Introduction to the Process of Nursing, Nursing of the Adult Adapting to Health Stressors I and II, Nursing of the Childbearing and Childrearing Family and Practicum, Family and Community Health Nursing and Practicum, Nursing Leadership and Practicum, Issues in Nursing, Research in Nursing, Mental Health Nursing, Nursing in the Community and Practicum	Chi Square, Structured Coefficient	Grades in an introductory nursing course taken during the sophomore year and in a medical-surgical nursing course taken during the junior year were substantially and directly related to NCLEX-RN performance. Grades earned in all other nursing theory courses had positive correlations with the discriminant function. Grades in the practicum courses were relatively poor predictors of NCLEX-RN performance

Author	Year	Purpose	Sample	Variables	Analysis	Findings
McKinney, J., Small, S., O'Dell, N., & Coonrod, B. A.	1988	To determine which measures of academic success, in a sample of 136 baccalaureate nursing graduates from a private liberal arts college between 1983 and 1985 predicted success on the National Council Licensing Examination (NCLEX)	136 baccalaureate nursing students	SAT Total, Math, Verbal; GPA; Mosby Assess Test Scores; NCLEX Scores; Age; Sex; Courses Repeated; Type A behavior	Multiple Regression and Pearson Product Moment ($p < .01-.001$)	Study concluded that nurse educators could identify students early in programs whose academic patterns suggest potential difficulty within the nursing major and likely failure on the NCLEX
Feldt, R. C., & Sister James Marie Donahue	1989	To identify the best linear combination of readily available scholastic variables, one set to predict success in a nursing program and the other to predict performance on the NCLEX-RN	155 students who completed and 34 who failed to complete a baccalaureate nursing program for the 1984–1986 years	GPA; ACT Composite Score; Chemistry Grade; Anatomy Grade; High School Percentile Rank	Multiple Regression, Chi Square, Correlation ($p < .001$)	The best set of predictors of nursing GPA included ACT composite score, anatomy grade and chemistry grade. The best set of predictors of NCLEX-RN included ACT composite score, high school percentile rank, nursing GPA and chemistry grade
Jenks, J., Selekman, J., Bross, T., & Paquet, M.	1989	To identify predictors of success in the NCLEX-RN and determine the optimal point in time for identifying students at risk	407 graduates of an integrated upper division baccalaureate nursing program from 1984–1987	Lower division GPA; Science GPA; Type of lower division college; Age; Sex; Junior level nursing course grades; Senior level nursing grades; Mosby Assess Test	Pearson Correlation Coefficient, Stepwise Regression Analysis ($p < .0001-01$)	Indication that students at high risk can be identified at the end of the junior year so that enrichment and support programs can be introduced at that time

(Continued)

Table 7.1 *Continued*

Author	Date	Purpose	Sample	Predictor Variables	Statistical Methods	Findings
Dell, M. S., & Valine, W. J.	1990	To determine multivariate relationships among collegiate GPA, SAT/ACT scores, self esteem and age in explaining differences in scores on the NCLEX-RN made by new graduates of baccalaureate nursing programs	90 senior generic nursing students in three small, 4 year public southeastern schools of nursing	GPA SAT/ACT Z Scores Self-Esteem Measures Age	Spearman-Brown Correlation, Multiple Regression, ($p < .001$)	GPA is one of the best predictors of success on national nursing examinations. There was a lack of contribution to the variance by the self-esteem measures
Lengacher, C. A., & Keller, R.	1990	To examine the relationship between selected admission variables, age, perception or role strain, achievement in clinical and nursing courses, achievement on NLN examinations, exit GPA and performance on NCLEX-RN examination	146 Associate degree graduates	Entrance GPA ACT sub-test Scores Age Perception of Role Strain Achievement in clinical and nursing courses Achievement on NLN examinations Exit GPA	Correlation coefficients, Stepwise Multiple Regression ($p < .001–.05$)	The best predictor of performance on the NCLEX-RN of the selected admission variables were exit GPA and ACT composite scores. The study findings indicate that nurse educators can identify students early in the program who would be successful on the NCLEX-RN and those who would be at risk for failure

Author	Year	Purpose	Sample	Variables	Analysis	Findings
Foti, L., & DeYoung, S.	1991	This retrospective correlational study was conducted to determine variables that predict success on the National Council Licensure Examination-Registered Nurse	296 nursing students that graduated between 1985 and 1988	GPA—overall GPA—in major GPA—in science SAT—verbal and quantitative NLN Baccalaureate Achievement Test Score Mosby Assess Test Score	Pearson Correlation and Multiple Regression Analysis (p < .0001)	Pearson correlations indicated the Mosby Assess Test, overall GPA and GPA in the major, NLN Achievement Test, and SAT verbal to be of moderate predictive value. Multiple regression analysis indicated that the most useful combination of predictors was the Mosby Assess Test, SAT verbal, and overall GPA
Horns, P. N., O'Sullivan, P., & Goodman, R.	1991	To determine predictors of success on the NCLEX preadmission and years 2, 3, and 4 variables in relation to NCLEX-RN scores	408 baccalaureate nursing students	Age Sex Race Admission GPA Grades for clinical courses Grades for clinical courses in mental health, adult health, and maternal child nursing Senior clinical course grades NLN comprehensive exam Graduate GPA	Forward Regression Analysis, Correlation Coefficients (p < .01)	Results suggest that there are preadmission and sophomore year predictors of NCLEX-RN success which could be used to design early interventions for students performing poorly and at risk of failing the NCLEX-RN

(Continued)

189

Table 7.1 *Continued*

Author	Date	Purpose	Sample	Predictor Variables	Statistical Methods	Findings
Poorman, S. G., & Martin, J.	1991	To determine the relationship of test anxiety, cognition, and general academic performance of second-semester senior level bachelor's degree students to success on the NCLEX	102 senior bachelor's degree nursing students	Test Anxiety Inventory Cognitive Assessment Tool Quality Point Average Student Aptitude Test scores	Multiple Regression, Pearson Product Moment Correlation, Chi Square ($p < .05$)	Research findings indicated that test anxiety was inversely related to passing score on the NCLEX. Academic aptitude positively correlated with passing scores on the NCLEX. Negative cognition were not inversely related to pass rate on the NCLEX. Self-perceived grades and self-predicted NCLEX scores were the best predictors of actual NCLEX scores. Subjects successful on the NCLEX were more likely to believe they were good test-takers and reported more facilitative thoughts during exams than those who failed the NCLEX
Fowles, E. R.	1992	To identify predictors of success on the NCLEX-RN and within the nursing curriculum	192 graduates of an upper division, single purpose baccalaureate nursing program	GPA ACT composite A & P grades Mosby Asses Test	Stepwise Multiple Regression Analysis, Correlation Coefficients ($p < .05$)	NCLEX success can be predicted and findings have implications for entering a nursing student into an early intervention program

Author	Year	Sample	Variables	Analysis	Findings
Mills, A. C., Sampel, M. E., Pohlman, V. C., & Becker, A. M.	1992	534 first time nurse candidates	Age Sex High School GPA Four sub-scores (social science, natural science, mathematics and English) Transfer Cumulative GPA for nursing courses at the end of each of the four academic years	Stepwise logistic regression, ($p < .05$)	Cumulative GPA suggested that the end of the sophomore year was the best time for predicting success and the end of the junior year was best for predicting failure. Age was inversely related to successful performance in three of the four models
Mills, A. C., Becker, A. M., Sampel, M. E., & Pohlman, V. C.	1992	328 first time nurse candidates for the NCLEX-RN from 1982 to 1990	Age Sex Education GPA Graduate work Cumulative semester GPAs	Logistic regression ($p < .05$)	The best time for predicting NCLEX-RN performance is at the end of an accelerated program

To identify academic predictors of success on the NCLEX-RN for nurse candidates who graduated from a four-year baccalaureate nursing program and to describe the odds for success of nurse candidates on their first attempt at the NCLEX-RN

To identify predictors of successful performance and determine probabilities of success on the NCLEX-RN

(Continued)

191

Table 7.1 *Continued*

Author	Date	Purpose	Sample	Predictor Variables	Statistical Methods	Findings
McClelland, E., Yang, J. C., & Glick, O. J.	1992	To validate, using a statewide sample, findings from two previous smaller investigations the relationships between admission selection variables and subsequent achievement in baccalaureate nursing programs and performance on the NCLEX-RN	1069 graduates of nine Iowa basic baccalaureate programs	Relationship between admission selection variables and subsequent achievement in the nursing program The extent to which achievement in nursing courses predicted performance on the NCLEX-RN Path analysis was used to formulate a causal model describing the relationships among the variables in the study	Pearson Product Moment Correlation Coefficients, Stepwise Multiple Regression ($p < .001–.01$)	Results suggest that students pre-nursing grade point average and American College testing scores predict their performance on the NCLEX-RN
Rami, S. J.	1992	To evaluate the importance of four predictor variables in predicting success on the NCLEX RN	35 graduates of a newly developed baccalaureate nursing program	Pre-Nursing GPA ACT Scores Comprehensive Examination Scores Basics I NLN Achievement Test	Multiple Regression Analysis, Pearson Product Moment ($p < .001–.05$)	Findings according to author are inconclusive. Basic I test scores were significantly correlated with successful achievement on the NCLEX-RN and were significant predictors of success. the Author recommends repeating the study with a larger sample

Author(s)	Year	Purpose	Sample	Variables	Analysis	Findings
Younger, J. B., & Grap, M. J.	1992	This study attempted to identify the best risk indices for students who do not pass NCLEX, to pinpoint the earliest time in their academic careers that their risk can substantially be known, and to estimate the effectiveness of a formal review course	388 graduates of an upper-division baccalaureate program who took the NCLEX examination between 1984 and 1987	Nursing school course grades Test scores of the Scholastic Aptitude Test National League for Nursing test scores	Correlation, Stepwise Multiple Regression	Nursing course grades, SAT scores, and NLN test scores can be used in combination to predict NCLEX performance. Whether a student took an NCLEX review course was not a significant predictor of performance
Frierson, H. T., Malone, B., & Shelton, P.	1993	The purpose of the study was to assess the associated effects of a three-pronged intervention procedure on NCLEX-RN performance	Eight African-American Nursing Students	The Three pronged approach consisted of: (1) instructions in effective test-taking, (2) participation in learning teams, (3) follow-up activities conducted by the faculty to reinforce the first two components	Correlation (p < .025)	The three pronged intervention effort was associated with a significantly improved NCLEX-RN passing rate and mean score (p. 224)

(Continued)

Table 7.1 *Continued*

Author	Date	Purpose	Sample	Predictor Variables	Statistical Methods	Findings
Wall, B. M., Miller, D. E., & Widerquist, J. G.	1993	To identify academic variables both before and during the nursing program that predict success or failure on NCLEX-RN and to determine how accurately students at risk of failure can be identified	92 graduates of an NLN accredited baccalaureate nursing program in a private, church affiliated liberal arts college in the Midwest	SAT High School Rank NLN Tests Mosby Assess Test	T-Test, Discriminant Function Analysis (p < .01–.15)	Findings indicate that data collected prior to entry in nursing program can be used to predict performance on current NCLEX-RN. Several variables were significantly better performance predictors and included: High School Rank, Sophomore GPA, GPA in sciences, nursing and Senior GPA, and NLN achievement tests taken at end of each nursing course
Waterhouse, J. K., Carroll, M. C., & Beeman, P. B.	1993	To identify variables that might be used as predictors for success on the post 1988 National Council Licensure Examination and to identify those students at risk of failing the examination	257 graduates of a baccalaureate nursing program from 1988 to 1990	15 variables examined SAT verbal SAT Math High School Percentile Physiology Grade Pathophysiology Grade Second Junior nursing course grade First senior nursing course grade Sophomore GPI Graduation GPI Last nursing clinical	Pearson Product Moment Correlation Coefficients (p < .05)	Findings indicate that reasonably accurate predictive data on individuals students performance is available by the end of the junior year, allowing faculty to begin interventions for at-risk students

| Heupel, C. | 1994 | To examine the relationship of selected academic variables to NCLEX-RN performance and determine a "best set" of indicators predictive of NCLEX-RN success | 152 basic students who completed the baccalaureate nursing program between 1985 and 1987 | Freshman Grade Point average
Sophomore Grade point average
Junior Grade Point Average
Senior Grade Point Average
Theory grades for five prerequisite science courses
Theory grades for three sophomore medical-surgical nursing courses
Theory grades for six junior medical-surgical and parent-child nursing courses
Theory grades for four senior mental health, community health, and leadership nursing courses | Multiple Regression Analysis and Pearson Product Moment Correlation Coefficients ($p < .0001–.05$) | The best predictors were a sophomore nursing theory course, a junior nursing theory course, the junior year grade point average, and a senior nursing theory course. Results of this study indicated that selected nursing theory courses and the JGPA could be used in a statistical model to predict pass or fail on the NCLEX-RN |

research regarding predictors of success on NCLEX-RN. Citations were tracked from one study to another. Every attempt was made to ensure a comprehensive review.

HISTORICAL SUMMARY OF LICENSURE EXAMINATION DEVELOPMENT

The examination to become licensed as a registered nurse has evolved and changed over time. Changes in the organization of the exam and the method of administration reflect changes in nursing curriculum designs, nursing practice, and the influence of technology. A brief overview of the most significant changes in format and administration of the exam serves to place the studies presented in some historical context while illuminating the impact of issues such as public safety and technology and the importance of these issues in terms of the examination's overall design and content.

The history of licensure was summarized by Matassarin-Jacobs (1989). She noted that prior to 1944, each state controlled its own licensure examination. In 1944, The National League for Nursing became involved in a nationwide testing program and established a test blueprint known as the State Board Test Pool Examination (SBTPE). By the early 1950s, all states were using the exam, setting their own passing score. In the middle to late 1950s, the American Nurses Association (ANA) became involved in the control of the examination while the National League for Nursing continued to administer it.

The National Council of State Boards of Nursing (NCSBN) assumed responsibility for licensure test development and administration in 1978 and continues to maintain this responsibility. A five-part content-based examination was initially developed with a passing score set yearly. A normative reference format was used (Matassarin-Jacobs, 1989).

In 1982, the examination was redesigned from normative referencing to criterion referencing and from a five-part format to a unified integrated test. The focus of the integration was the nursing process and included eight areas of human functioning. The overall passing score was set at 1600 (Matassarin-Jacobs, 1989).

After July 1988, the examination scoring was changed to pass/fail. Nursing process continued to be the basis for the overall design of the examination in addition to four areas of client needs that included safety, physiologic integrity, psychosocial integrity, and health promotion. The examination continues to be criterion referenced (Matassarin-Jacobs, 1989).

Scoring changes to pass/fail had far reaching effects. According to Washburn and Short (1992), student preparation for and performance on the pass/fail examination were affected by these scoring changes. In their study, nursing education administrators were surveyed regarding their "knowledge of NCLEX-RN changes, their opinions regarding the changes, and their involvement in the change process" (p. 17). Approximately three-fourths of the administrators (75.8% BSN and 71.4% ADN) reported that they were not well informed (p. 172).

The original random study sample included 100 administrators of baccalaureate nursing programs (BSN) and 100 administrators of associate degree nursing programs (ADN) for a total of 200. The response rate was 60% ($n = 120$) with approximately half of the respondents from the baccalaureate program and half from the associate degree program. The tool had been pilot tested using 10 nursing program administrators randomly selected from BSN and ADN programs and was reviewed for content validity and clarity. Since the overall response rate was above 50% on the mailed questionnaire and the sample was randomly chosen, one can have confidence in the validity of these findings.

According to the National Council of State Boards of Nursing (1990), difficulty of test items and the number of test items had no effect on the passing rate. This is due to the fact that the passing standards on the NCLEX are criterion referenced which means "the standard is referenced to the content and difficulty of test items, as opposed to a norm-referenced approach, in which the standard is referenced to the performance of a normative group of examinees" (NCSBN, 1990, p. 10). A change in the passing standard will effect a change in the passing rate unless the level of candidate competence (ability to practice entry-level nursing safely and effectively as measured by the NCLEX) changes. "Effective with the July, 1988 examination, the RN passing standard was increased slightly, so that candidates had to answer approximately three more items correctly in order to pass the examination. This increase, and a simultaneous drop in the NCLEX-estimated competence level of candidates taking the July, 1988 examination was associated with a drop in the passing rate of approximately eight percentage points" (Matassarin-Jacobs, 1989, p. 12).

In the late 1980s, the National Council of State Boards of Nursing (NCSBN) devoted considerable time, money, and effort in the development of computerized adaptive testing (CAT). Field tests for computerized adaptive testing were conducted in July 1990 and February 1991. The purpose was to determine the feasibility of using a CAT mode for administering licensure tests by studying the efficiency, measurement properties, logistics, and costs. Analysis of the data from these field trials showed that CAT gave comparable measurement of candidates' performance as with the previous paper-and-pencil type of administration. It was also determined that neither demographics nor prior computer experience had any effect on performance. In addition, the

CAT was determined to be psychometrically sound (NCSBN, 1993, p. 11). CAT is based on the principle that for each examinee, some questions will be more effective than others in revealing levels of competence. As the candidate answers each question, the computer calculates a competence level.

National implementation of this examination method, which is based on a psychometric model known as Item Response Theory (IRT) was initiated by NCSBN in July 1994. "The central concept of IRT is the item characteristic curve (ICC), a function that represents the probability of answering a given item correctly given an examinee's latent trait or ability. It is assumed that as ability increases, so does the probability of answering an item correctly" (Halkitis & Leahy, 1993, p. 380).

This method of testing presents both students and faculty with new challenges for the teaching-learning process. These challenges include ensuring that students are comfortable using computerized testing and developing critical thinking skills that promote sound decision making and problem solving in clinical situations. The student will benefit from the fact that the test will be structured for the individual and administered more frequently. Other benefits include the fact that the test will not pass marginal candidates, thus improving the protection of the public, it will lessen or eliminate the need for temporary permits and will help to alleviate supply problems by providing more immediate results, thus putting new nurses in the mainstream of the workplace more quickly (NCSBN, 1989).

A future step into technology is being studied by the NCSBN in its work toward a computerized Clinical Simulation Test (CST) of nursing competence. The intent of this project is to address performance assessment concerns that paper-and-pencil examinations are not capable of evaluating. Competence to practice professional nursing would be better evaluated using a simulated type testing procedure which would require the use of decision-making and problem-solving skills. Based on the nursing process, the examinee is given a case study and then must proceed with data gathering and intervention activities (NCSBN, 1993, p. 1). The client responds to these activities as the examinee moves through the simulation. Study of this project will continue through 1997 and "at the completion of this phase, a decision will be made by the National Council membership regarding the future use of CST" (NCSBN, 1993, p. 8).

THE LICENSURE EXAMINATION: HOW VALID IS IT?

The purpose of licensure is to ensure that professional nursing provides competent, safe nursing care to the public. The licensure examination is currently our only measurement for minimum safe practice and therefore must be a valid and reliable measure of the knowledge required to practice professional nursing.

Kane (1982) further addressed issues of validity on professional licensure examinations. He addressed issues surrounding content validity and how this might be ascertained. One suggestion included having a committee of experienced practitioners or "experts" decide which nursing competencies need to be evaluated.

Kane (1982) suggested that using direct observation and/or asking practitioners how they spend their working hours are two ways to determine what goes on in practice, providing data on the kinds of demands placed on practitioners. "The major difficulty with studies of how professionals spend their time is that many of the activities that appear in the results of the studies may not involve service to clients, and therefore may not be closely related to the purpose of licensure—protection of the public" (Kane, 1982, p. 912). Questioning the validity of licensure examinations is critical if we are to do what we promise with the exam, ensure public safety. The CST, should it be incorporated into the licensure exam, would address the concerns expressed by Kane.

Froman and Owen (1989) questioned the validity of the changed licensure examination from the State Board Examination to that developed by the NCSBN (NCLEX). Although the emphasis on the nursing process as the model of care seemed appropriate for testing, the authors cited the sparsity of evidence in regard to concurrent, predictive, or construct validity both for the SBE and NCLEX (p. 334). Also to be considered is the fact that the licensure examination still does not differentiate between diploma, associate, and baccalaureate degree programs.

According to the NCSBN (1993), job analysis is an essential first step in the development of NCLEX. "The validity of a licensure examination (such as NCLEX) rests squarely on the relationship of the examination to safe and effective practice. The primary focus of the relationship to practice is the examination's job analysis based on content validity. NCLEX administered by CAT is clearly valid from this perspective" (NCSBN, 1993, p. 6).

Job analysis is conducted every three years and involves data collection of nursing activities performed by a stratified random sample of over 3,000 newly licensed nurses. Nursing activities are rated regarding frequency and criticality of each activity. The data are submitted to statistical testing and along with expert judgment the test plan is reviewed and revised. Item development is then implemented through NCLEX development panels. Item writers are selected, trained, and assisted in the development of the examination. The minimum standard or passing point is reviewed by a panel of judges every three years. Changes in the passing point are made as necessary (Campbell-Warnock, Jones-Dickson, & Fields, 1993).

PREDICTORS OF SUCCESS IN BACCALAUREATE, ASSOCIATE, AND DIPLOMA NURSING PROGRAMS

Predicting success on the NCLEX-RN has always been a concern of nurse educators in diploma, associate, and baccalaureate programs. Predictors are those factors that provide the best measure of a student's ability to succeed on the licensure examination. Some predictors may be very program-specific, such as grades in science courses or nursing courses. Other predictors used are more standardized measures such as NLN Achievement exams and the Mosby Assess Test. Each program must evaluate on an individual basis the variables which will best predict their graduates' success on the licensure examination. The review that follows emphasizes those variables which have had the most predictive value for baccalaureate, associate, and diploma programs and can provide direction for others initiating such studies.

Baccalaureate Programs

A number of research studies addressing predictors of success in baccalaureate nursing programs have focused on pre-admission criteria as indicators of success on NCLEX-RN. High school GPA and subscales of the American College Testing Exam (ACT) are two predictor variables that have been utilized in numerous studies. Mills, Sampel, Pohlman, and Becker (1992), in their study of 534 nurse candidates for the NCLEX-RN from 1982 to 1990 utilized stepwise logistic regression as the multivariate technique and found the admission variables of GPA and ACT scores to be weak predictors of examination performance. Logistic regression was appropriate since it does not require the assumption of a normal distribution for NCLEX pass rates or the multivariate normality of GPA and ACT scores. However, several studies found the admission GPA to be useful in predicting successful performance on the NCLEX-RN (Friedemann & Valentine, 1988; Horns, O'Sullivan, & Goodman, 1991; Payne & Duffey, 1986; Sharp, 1984; Stronck, 1979; Yocom & Scherubel, 1985). All of the previous authors used stepwise multiple regression in their analysis of admission GPA and performance on NCLEX except for Horns, O'Sullivan, and Goodman (1991) who used a forward regression procedure. Given that the same model for regression was used in the majority of the referenced studies, the results are more reliable in prediction of NCLEX success. GPA and ACT scores appear to be valid variables to be used in the prediction of success on NCLEX at the completion of a baccalaureate nursing program.

Yang, Glick, and McClelland (1987) included high school rank as a variable and found a direct correlation with NCLEX-RN scores and ACT Social Science subscores. SAT and ACT subscale scores have also been investigated as predictors of performance on the NCLEX-RN. Some studies have found the verbal and social science scores to be high predictors of performance (Foti & DeYoung, 1991; McClelland, Yang, & Glick, 1992; McKinney, Small, O'Dell, & Coonrod, 1988; Payne & Duffey, 1986; Perez, 1977; Quick, Krupa, & Whitley, 1985; Sharp, 1984; Yang, Glick, & McClelland, 1987). However, Dell and Valine (1990) found "the SAT/ACT scores added nothing significant to the explanation of the variance of the NCLEX-RN scores beyond that of GPA" (p. 161). In this study, both GPA and SAT/ACT scores were highly correlated which resulted in the finding that SAT/ACT scores did not significantly add to the variance of the NCLEX-RN scores beyond that of the GPA.

A number of studies included variations of the GPA as predictors of NCLEX success. Sharp (1984), Payne and Duffey (1986), and Glick, McClelland, and Yang (1986) found that math and natural science GPAs had predictive value. Cumulative GPAs at various points throughout the four years of a baccalaureate program were found to strengthen prediction for passing the licensure examination (Foti & DeYoung, 1991; Horns, O'Sullivan, & Goodman, 1991; Mills, Becker, Sampel, & Pohlman, 1992; Mills, Sampel, Pohlman, & Becker, 1992; Sr. St. Thomas, 1982). Marquis and Worth (1992) utilized descriptive statistics and Pearson Correlation Coefficients as well as varimax rotated factor analysis. These authors reported nursing GPA, non-nursing GPA, and faculty clinical evaluations (Likert Scale Grading 1 = poor and 5 = superior) of students during their eight clinical rotations to be correlated with passing NCLEX scores. The authors found these three factors to be closely related, although the nursing GPA and non-nursing GPA most closely defined the predictive factor.

There are a variety of factors to consider when examining GPA and specific courses in terms of their value in predicting success on the NCLEX-RN. Although each baccalaureate program has similar goals, specific course work in general education and nursing will vary. These variations will no doubt influence their value as predictors of NCLEX success. Therefore, it would seem that each program must evaluate these variables on an individual basis. They will not have the same predictive value for all baccalaureate programs.

The NLN test scores were used as predictors in numerous studies. Bell and Martindill (1976) found the NLN scores for Nursing of Children and Obstetric Nursing to be indicators of SBE success and Melcolm and Bausell (1981) reported all NLN achievement tests as having predictive value. Foti and DeYoung (1991) and Younger and Grap (1992) reported the NLN Baccalaureate Achievement test to have a high correlation with NCLEX success. Rami (1992) found that NLN Basic I Test Scores correlated with NCLEX success.

More recent studies have used the Mosby Assess Test as a predictor of NCLEX and have reported positive correlations (Foti & DeYoung, 1991; Jenks, Selekman, Bross, & Paquet, 1989; McKinney, Small, O'Dell, &

Coonrod, 1988). The NLN Achievement tests and Mosby Assess Test are standardized examinations and are therefore more consistent and reliable in terms of their ability to predict success on the NCLEX-RN. The varied use of Pearson correlations and multiple regression techniques in the NLN examinations and Mosby Assess Test studies consistently evaluated these methods as positive predictors of NCLEX success.

Ashley (1990) studied the effects of three NCLEX preparation programs on nursing knowledge test anxiety and licensure examination performance. All subjects achieved high scores on a nursing achievement test and showed slight reduction in overall test anxiety. No statistical differences were found for the NCLEX passing rates of the three groups.

Sheil and Meisenheimer (1992) reported a research study using a 2-day anxiety reducing workshop with a mixed group of new graduates in an acute care setting. All subjects experienced a reduction in anxiety as measured by Zung's Self-Rating Anxiety Scale and all participants passed the NCLEX-RN examination.

Studies addressing test anxiety are important since student test anxiety can be an important factor in their ability to succeed on the examination. Identifying test anxiety early in the students' academic career can offer students opportunity to master test-taking skills while at the same time mastering content.

Zink (1991) conducted a retrospective study of 236 baccalaureate graduates from a single university and found:

1. Pre-nursing GPA is a good predictor of success/nonsuccess on the NCLEX-RN.
2. Science course GPAs are positively correlated to performance on the NCLEX-RN.
3. Students' cumulative nursing course GPAs show a positive correlation to NCLEX-RN performance.
4. Nursing courses in the junior and senior year show a direct correlation with performance on the NCLEX-RN (pp. 64–65).

A study of 384 graduates of a BSN program who took the NCLEX-RN during the years of 1982 through 1985 was conducted by Krupa, Quick, and Whitley (1988). Grades for an introductory nursing course and a junior level nursing course were found to be related to successful NCLEX-RN performance. The investigators concluded: "grades in nursing courses hold a great deal of promise as predictors of performance on the NCLEX-RN" (p. 297). Friedemann and Valentine (1988) also found nursing lecture course grades to be better predictors of NCLEX success than clinical courses. In addition, Younger and Grap (1992) found nursing school course grades in combination with SAT scores and

NLN test scores to predict NCLEX success. Heupel's study (1994) of 152 basic baccalaureate students described the best predictors of NCLEX success to be a sophomore and junior nursing theory course, the junior year grade point average and a senior nursing theory course.

Waterhouse, Carroll, and Beeman (1993), in a study of 257 graduates from one program during the years of 1988–1990, found the two best predictors of NCLEX success to be the first senior-level nursing course grade and the graduation grade-point index. In addition, accurate prediction data were compiled on 86% of the students by the end of their junior year of study and this gradually increased to 91% by the time of graduation.

Results on the latest NCLEX-RN initiated in 1988 were studied by Wall, Miller, and Widerquist (1993). Findings suggested similarities regarding predictors among this latest NCLEX (pass/fail score) and the prior one (numerical score). The high school rank, pre-nursing science and sophomore GPAs were found to be positive predictors. In addition, NLN Achievement test scores, nursing GPA, and the Mosby Assess Test score were significant predictors of NCLEX performance for this group of 92 graduates from the 1988–1991 classes of a baccalaureate nursing program.

Nonacademic variables have also been found to affect NCLEX success rates. Poorman and Martin (1991) reported test anxiety to be inversely related to passing scores on NCLEX and the "best predictors of actual NCLEX performance were self-predicted NCLEX scores and self-perceived grades [not actual GPA but the letter grade that the students believed best described their performance]" (p. 30). Ashley and O'Neil (1991) described a long-term intervention program consisting of test-coaching, and test-taking skills to be effective for at-risk students in passing the NCLEX-RN.

Associate Degree Nursing Programs

Deardorff, Denner, and Miller (1976) studied graduates from one associate degree nursing program between the years of 1969-1974. Multiple regression and correlation analysis was used to compare performance on NLN achievement tests with scores on the State Board Examination. The specific achievement test of Sick Children, Medical Nursing, and Postpartum, were found to predict state board examination scores (p. 38). Aldag and Rose (1983) examined a sample of 787 students admitted to an associate degree program over a span of 10 years. Two groups comprised the sample: 555 traditional students who were admitted based on high school rank and composite scores on the ACT or equivalent and 232 nontraditional students admitted based on obtaining a 2.00 GPA after completing 18 semester hours in the college.

All interval data were analyzed with the ANOVA and Pearson Product Moment techniques and the level of significance was set at $p < .01$. Results of the study pointed to a negative age bias on the ACT. In addition, a larger proportion of the older students graduate and initially pass State Boards than the proportion of the younger group (p. 71). "No significant differences were found between the traditional and nontraditional admissions for graduation rate or initial pass rate for the State Board" (p. 71). However age was "positively related to performance on the State Board examinations" (p. 73) and for this sample of associate degree students, the nontraditional admission criteria (2.00 GPA and 18-hour program of study in the college instead of high school rank and ACT scores) proved to be predictive.

Woodham and Taube (1986) examined three graduating classes from an Associate degree program. Seven required nursing courses, SAT verbal, and math scores, age at graduation and high school class rank were chosen as predictor variables. All seven nursing courses and SAT verbal scores had a significant positive relationship with passing NCLEX ($p = < .01$) (p. 115). Lengacher and Keller (1990) examined multiple admission variables (entrance GPA, ACT scores in English and Math and composite ACT scores), age, perception of role strain, achievement in clinical and nursing courses, NLN examination scores, exit GPA, and performance on NCLEX-RN among 146 graduates who wrote the exam in 1987 and 1988. The best predictors were found to be the exit GPA, ACT composite scores, two nursing theory courses in the second year of the program and the Basic Two and Psychiatric NLN examinations (p. 163). Similar findings by Felts (1986) have been reported. Data analysis of 297 first time writers of the NCLEX-RN between 1982 and 1984 reveal the ACT composite score to be the best admission criteria predictor for success in nursing courses and the overall college performance predicts pass/fail status on the NCLEX-RN better than high school criteria. Grades in the sciences and the humanities differentiated students who passed and failed NCLEX. Age and licensure as an LPN did not predict NCLEX performance.

Breyer (1984) studied a sample of 511 associate degree graduates and 350 diploma graduates and found "a strong relationship between success on the Comprehensive Nursing Achievement Test and success on the Nurse Licensure Examination" (p. 194). Cloud-Hardaway (1988) conducted an ex post facto study of 558 Associate Degree Nursing graduates who wrote the NCLEX in 1983 and 1984. Significant relationships were found among the Mosby Assess Test scores and semester averages and success on NCLEX.

Variables examined to predict success on the licensure examination for graduates of associate degree programs are similar to those used in baccalaureate programs. Since associate degree programs have a greater tendency to attract nontraditional students (older students, second career students, students with families), different personality factors must be taken into consideration when attempting to predict performance on the licensure examination. For example, the fact that students may be older, more mature, and have responsibilities such as work and home must be taken into consideration.

Diploma Nursing Programs

Washburn (1980) conducted a study of 166 graduates of a diploma program between the years of 1976 and 1978. She found a significant correlation between the NLN Achievement tests (Nursing Care of Patients I, II, and III; Obstetric Nursing; Psychiatric Nursing and Nursing of Children) and State Board Test Pool Examination results. Results of Breyer's study (1984) of 2,496 associate degree and diploma students supported the NLN Comprehensive Nursing Achievement test as a predictor of NCLEX-RN performance.

Two studies have focused on critical thinking and predictors of success in a nursing program. Gross, Takazawa, and Rose (1987) found improvement in critical thinking as measured by the Watson-Glaser Critical Thinking Appraisal scale to have improved over the four years but was not of itself predictive of NCLEX success. NCLEX was best predicted by the GPA. Bauwens and Gerhard (1987) found the Watson-Glaser Critical Thinking Appraisal to be useful as a pre-admission predictor of nursing success. Critical thinking skills are necessary to ensure sound decision-making and problem-solving skills in clinical situations. The emphasis placed on critical thinking by the National League for Nursing further supports the need for developing these skills in graduates of nursing programs. The next step is to measure these skills and examine them in terms of their ability to predict success on the licensure examination.

SPECIAL NEEDS OF MINORITY STUDENTS

Several researchers looked specifically at minority students and what might be useful in prediction of success on the NCLEX-RN examination. Outtz (1979) found that high school GPA correlated with college GPA and that SAT scores had a high correlation with State Board Test Pool Examination (SBTPE) scores. The cumulative college GPA was the best predictor with the SAT verbal component the second best predictor of success on the license examination. A later study by Dell and Halpin (1984) found the senior year GPA, SAT verbal component, and the NLN pre-nursing test to be the best predictors of success. Boyle

(1986) compared two minority groups, blacks and non-blacks, and discovered the entering grade point average and American College Test Assessment (ACT) to be the best predictors of success with ACT the strongest and best predictor. Crane, Wright, and Michael (1987) studied predictor variables for a group of 418 mixed minority students seeking a diploma in nursing. The subject group included Hispanics, Blacks, Asians, and Whites. For the White and Hispanic groups, the nursing courses' grade point average were the most valid predictor of NCLEX success and selected NLN Achievement tests gave higher predictive validity for the Black and Asian groups. Students who took courses in the community college prior to entering the program tended to achieve higher GPAs in their nursing courses but there was little predictive validity for the NCLEX-RN based on this variable. The NLN Achievement tests proved to be positive predictors for both nursing course GPA and success on NCLEX-RN.

SUMMARY

Many similarities exist among diploma, associate, and baccalaureate degree nursing programs regarding predictors of success on the licensure examination. Pre-admission criteria such as high school grade-point average, American College Test (ACT), Scholastic Aptitude Test (SAT-verbal/math), and high school rank (HSR) were found in various combinations to have some correlation with success on the NCLEX-RN. Many of the studies found the National League for Nursing test scores (NLN) in combination with specific nursing theory courses to be the best predictors of NCLEX success. Of particular interest is the finding that clinical nursing course grades were not predictive of passing NCLEX. This is most probably due to the fact that clinical performance is more difficult to measure objectively, and faculty use various methods of grading performance, i.e., satisfactory/unsatisfactory, pass/fail, numerical, and/or letter grades. In contrast, theory courses are more standardized regarding measurement of knowledge and offer more objective information regarding students' abilities.

The NLN Baccalaureate Achievement test and the Mosby Assess Test have been predictive for the majority of programs. It appears the key to predictive power of these criteria is the model of combination that is used. Some studies reported the combination of Mosby Assess Test and Nursing GPA as better predictors than the NLN Achievement tests and nursing theory courses. Some specific combinations that have been reported in the literature are: nursing GPA, non-nursing GPA, and faculty clinical evaluations; nursing course grades, SAT scores and the NLN Achievement tests; high school rank, pre-nursing science grades, and the sophomore GPA; NLN Achievement tests, nursing GPA, and the Mosby Assess Test. The combination of predictor variables differs from one program to the next. This may be due to factors such as curricular design, characteristics of the student body and/or the faculty.

Numerous studies have been conducted as nursing education programs attempt to identify students at risk for failing the licensure examination and ultimately intervene to assist the student in preparing for and succeeding on the examination. Issues that need to be given consideration include the organization of the curriculum, program type, background of faculty teaching the major nursing/clinical courses and the composition of the student body. Each program is unique, taking different paths to achieve the same end—successful performance on the NCLEX-RN. This review offers the reader an opportunity to review those variables that have had the most success in predicting success on the NCLEX-RN as well as those variables that were less likely to predict success. Ultimately, each program needs to identify which variables provide the most accurate prediction of success for their own students, given the uniqueness of each program.

REFERENCES

Aldag, J., & Rose, S. (1983). Relationship of age, American College testing scores, grade point average and state board examination scores. *Research in Nursing & Health, 6*(2), 69–73.

Ashley, J. E. (1990). *The effects of three NCLEX preparation programs on nursing knowledge, on test anxiety, and on registered nurse licensure examination performance.* Unpublished Doctoral Dissertation. Boston College: Boston.

Ashley, J., & O'Neil, J. (1991). The effectiveness of an intervention to promote successful performance on NCLEX-RN for baccalaureate students at risk for failure. *Journal of Nursing Education, 30*(8), 360–366.

Bauwens, E. E., & Gerhard, G. G. (1987). The use of the Watson-Glaser critical thinking appraisal to predict success in a baccalaureate nursing program. *Journal of Nursing Education, 26*(7), 278–281.

Bell, J. A., & Martindill, C. F. (1976). A cross-validation study for predictors of scores on state board examinations. *Nursing Research, 25*(1), 54–57.

Boyle, K. K. (1986). Predicting the success of minority students in a baccalaureate nursing program. *Journal of Nursing Education, 25*(5), 186–192.

Breyer, F. J. (1984). The comprehensive nursing achievement test as a predictor of performance on the NCLEX-RN. *Nursing and Health Care,* April, 193–195.

Campbell-Warnock, J., Jones-Dickson, C., & Fields, F. (1993). The NCLEX development process: Some things don't change. *Issues, 5,* 6, 8, 9, 10.

Cloud-Hardaway, S. A. (1988). *Relationship among "Mosby's Assess Test" scores, academic performance, and demographic factors and associate degree nursing graduates NCLEX scores.* Unpublished doctoral dissertation, North Texas State University, Denton, Texas.

Crane, P., Wright, C. R., & Michael, W. B. (1987). School-related variables as predictors of achievement on the national council licensure examination (NCLEX-RN) for a sample of 418 students enrolled in a diploma nursing program. *Educational and Psychological Measurement,* 1055–1069.

Deardorff, M., Denner, P., & Miller, C. (1976). Selected National League of Nursing achievement test scores as predictors of state board examination scores. *Nursing Research, 25*(1), 35–38.

Dell, M. A., & Halpin, G. (1984). Predictors of success in nursing school and on state board examinations in a predominantly black baccalaureate nursing program. *Journal of Nursing Education, 23*(4), 147–150.

Dell, M. S., & Valine, W. J. (1990). Explaining differences in NCLEX-RN scores with certain cognitive and non-cognitive factors for new baccalaureate nurse graduates. *Journal of Nursing Education, 29*(4), 158–162.

Feldt, R. C., & Donahue, J. M. (1989). Predicting nursing GPA and National Council Licensure Examination for Registered Nurses (NCLEX-RN): A thorough analysis. *Psychological Reports, 64*(2), 415–421.

Felts, J. (1986). Performance predictors for nursing courses and NCLEX-RN. *Journal of Nursing Education, 25*(9), 372–377.

Foti, I., & DeYoung, S. (1991). Predicting success on the national council licensure examination-registered nurse: Another piece of the puzzle. *Journal of Professional Nursing, 7*(2), 99–104.

Fowles, E. R. (1992). Predictors of success on NCLEX-RN and within the nursing curriculum: Implications for early intervention. *Journal of Nursing Education, 31*(2), 53–57.

Friedemann, M. L., & Valentine, S. (1988). Success in old and new licensure examinations: Pre-admission factors and academic performance. *Research in Nursing and Health, 11,* 343–350.

Frierson, H. H., Malone, B., & Shelton, P. (1993). Enhancing NCLEX-RN performance: Assessing a three-pronged intervention approach. *Journal of Nursing Education, 35*(5), 222–224.

Froman, R. D., & Owen, S. V. (1989). Predicting performance on the National Council Licensure Examination. *Western Journal of Nursing Research, 11*(3), 334–346.

Glick, O. J., McClelland, E., & Yang, J. C. (1986). NCLEX-RN: Predicting the performance of graduates of an integrated baccalaureate nursing program. *Journal of Professional nursing, 2,* 98–103.

Gross, Y. T., Takazawa, E. S., & Rose, C. L. (1987). Critical thinking and nursing education. *Journal of Nursing Education, 26*(8), 317–323.

Halkitis, P. N., & Leahy, J. M. (1993). Computerized adaptive testing: The future is upon us. *Nursing and Health Care, 14*(7), 378–385.

Heupel, C. (1994). A model for intervention and predicting success on the national council licensure examination for registered nurses. *Journal of Professional Nursing, 10*(1), 57–60.

Horns, P. N., O'Sullivan, P., & Goodman, R. (1991). The use of progressive indicators as predictors of NCLEX-RN success and performance of BSN graduates. *Journal of Nursing Education, 30*(1), 9–14.

Jenks, J., Selekman, J., Bross, T., & Paquet, M. (1989). Success in NCLEX-RN: Identifying predictors and optimal timing for intervention. *Journal of Nursing Education, 28*(3), 112–118.

Kane, M. T. (1982). The validity of licensure examinations. *American Psychologist, 37*(8), 911–918.

Krupa, K. C., Quick, M. M., & Whitley, T. W. (1988). The effectiveness of nursing grades in predicting performance on the NCLEX-RN. *Journal of Professional Nursing, 4*(4), 294–298.

Lengacher, C. A., & Keller, R. (1990). Academic predictors of success on the NCLEX-RN examination for Registered Nurses. *Journal of Nursing Education, 29*(4), 163–169.

Marquis, B., & Worth, C. (1992). The relationship among multiple assessments of nursing education outcomes. *Journal of Nursing Education, 31*(1), 33–38.

Matassarin-Jacobs, E. (1989). The nursing licensure process and the NCLEX-RN. *Nurse Educator, 14*(6), 32–35.

McClelland, E., Yang, J. C., & Glick, O. J. (1992). A statewide study of academic variables affecting performance of baccalaureate nursing graduates on licensure examination. *Journal of Professional Nursing, 8*(6), 342–350.

McKinney, J., Small, S., O'Dell, N., & Coonrod, B. A. (1988). Identification of predictors of success for the NCLEX and students at risk for NCLEX failure in a baccalaureate nursing program. *Journal of Professional Nursing, 4,* 55–59.

Melcolm, N., & Bausell, R. B. (1981). The prediction of state board test pool examinations scores within an integrated curriculum. *Journal of Nursing Education, 20*(5), 24–28.

Mills, A. C., Becker, A. M., Sampel, M. E., & Pohlman, V. C. (1992). Success-failure on the national council licensure examination for registered nurses by nurse candidates from an accelerated baccalaureate nursing program. *Journal of Professional Nursing, 8*(6), 351–357.

Mills, A. C., Sampel, M. E., Pohlman, V. C., & Becker, A. M. (1992). The odds for success on NCLEX-RN by nurse candidates from a four-year baccalaureate nursing program. *Journal of Nursing Education, 31*(9), 403–408.

National Council of State Boards of Nursing, Inc. (1989). 1990 Marks start of field testing for computerized adaptive testing project. *Issues, 10*(4), 2, 4.

National Council of State Boards of Nursing, Inc. (1990). What affects NCLEX passing rates? *Issues, 11*(4), 10–15.

National Council of State Boards of Nursing, Inc. (1993a). Field tests of NCLEX using computerized adaptive testing. *Issues,* (special edition), 7, 11, 14.

National Council of State Boards of Nursing, Inc. (1993b). A new generation in competence assessment in nursing: Computerized clinical simulation test (CST). *Issues, 14*(1), 1–8.

Outtz, J. H. (1979). Predicting the success on state board examinations for blacks. *Journal of Nursing Education, 18*(9), 35–40.

Payne, M. A., & Duffey, M. A. (1986). An investigation of the predictability of NCLEX scores of BSN graduates using academic predictors. *Journal of Professional Nursing, 2,* 326–332.

Perez, T. L. (1977). Investigation of academic moderator variables to predict success on state board of nursing examinations in a baccalaureate nursing program. *Journal of Nursing Education, 16*(8), 16–23.

Poorman, S. G., & Martin, J. (1991). The role of nonacademic variables in passing the national council licensure examination. *Journal of Professional Nursing, 7*(1), 25–32.

Quick, M. M., Krupa, K. C., & Whitley, T. W. (1985). Using admission data to predict success on the NCLEX-RN in a baccalaureate program. *Journal of Professional Nursing, 1,* 364–368.

Rami, J. S. (1992). Predicting nursing students' success on NCLEX-RN. *ABNF-Journal, 3*(3), 67–71.

Schwirian, P. M., Baer, C. L., Basta, S. M., & Larabee, J. G. (1978). *Prediction of successful nursing performance.* Pub. No. 0-245-048, U.S. Government Printing Office.

Sharp, T. G. (1984). An analysis of the relationship of seven selected variables to state board test pool examination performance of the University of Tennessee, Knoxville, College of Nursing. *Journal of Nursing Education, 23*(2), 57–63.

Sheil, E. P., & Meisenheimer, C. G. (1992). Helping new graduates succeed at the NCLEX-RN experience, Evaluation of an Anxiety-reducing workshop. *Journal of Nursing Staff Development, 8*(5), 213–217.

Stronck, D. R. (1979). Predicting student performance from college admission criteria. *Nursing Outlook, 27*(9), 604–607.

St. Thomas, S. (1982). *An analysis of the relationship between the first semester grade point average and the state board nursing scores of Vermont college graduates.* Unpublished paper, Nova University.

Taylor, C. W., Nahm, H., Quinn, M., Harms, M., Mulaik, J., & Mulaik, S. A. (1965). *Report of Measurement and Predication of Nursing Performance, Part I.* University of Utah, Salt Lake City.

Taylor. C. W., Nahm. H., Loy, L., Harms, M., Berthod, J., & Wolfer, J. A. (1966). *Selection and recruitment of nurses and nursing students.* University of Utah Press, Salt Lake City.

Wagner, L., Henry, B., Giovinco, G., & Banks, C. (1988). Suggestions for graduate education in nursing service administration. *Journal of Nursing Education, 27*(5), 210–218.

Wall, B. M., Miller, D. E., & Widerquist, J. G. (1993). Predictors of success on the newest NCLEX-RN. *Western Journal of Nursing Research, 15*(5), 628–643.

Washburn, J. (1980). *Relationship of achievement test scores and state board performance in a diploma nursing program.* Indiana University at South Bend. EDRS-ED 203572, Doctoral Dissertation.

Washburn, J., & Short, L. (1992). The NCLEX-RN and nurse educators. *Journal of Nursing Education, 31*(4), 171–174.

Waterhouse, J. K., Carroll, M. C., & Beeman, P. B. (1993). National council licensure examination success: Accurate prediction of student performance on the post-1988 examination. *Journal of Professional Nursing, 9*(5), 278–283.

Woodham, R., & Taube, K. (1986). Relationship of nursing program predictors and success on the NCLEX-RN examination for licensure in a selected associate degree program. *Journal of Nursing Education, 25*(3), 112–117.

Yang, J. C., Glick, O. J., & McClelland, E. (1987). Academic correlates of baccalaureate graduate performance on NCLEX-RN. *Journal of Professional Nursing, 3,* 298–306.

Yocom, C. J., & Scherubel, J. C. (1985). Selected pre-admission and academic correlates of success on state board examinations. *Journal of Nursing Education, 24*(6), 244–249.

Younger, J. B., & Grap, M. J. (1992). An epidemiologic study of NCLEX. *Nurse Educator, 17*(2), 24–28.

Zink, M. H. (1991). *Performance of at-risk students of a baccalaureate degree nursing program in selected nursing courses and on the national council licensure examination for registered nurses.* Unpublished Doctoral Dissertation, Ball State University, Indiana.

aav-9830